Leslie Klenerman and Bernard Wood

The Human Foot

A Companion to Clinical Studies

With 85 Figures

With contribution by: Nicole L. Griffin, MS
Hominid Paleobiology Doctoral Program
George Washington University
Washington DC, USA

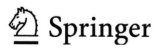 Springer

Leslie Klenerman, MBBCh, ChM, FRCS
Emeritus Professor of Orthopaedic
and Accident Surgery, The University of Liverpool,
Liverpool, UK

Bernard Wood, MBBS, PhD, DSc
Henry R. Luce Professor of Human Origins, Center
for the Advanced Study of Hominid Paleobiology,
Department of Anthropology, George Washington
University, Washington DC, USA

A catalogue record for this book is available from the British Library

Library of Congress Control Number: 2005925191

ISBN-10: 1-85233-925-X   Printed on acid-free paper
ISBN-13: 978-1-85233-925-8

Printed in the United States of America.   (SPI/EB)

9 8 7 6 5 4 3 2 1

Springer Science+Business Media
springeronline.com

Royal Liverpool University Hospital – Staff Library (Education Centre)

Please return or renew, on or before the last date below. A fine is payable on late returned items. Books may be recalled after one week for the use of another reader. Books may be renewed by telephone : 0151-706-2248

The Human Foot

Preface

The appendages at the end of our forelimbs tend to attract the evolutionary and clinical limelight, but our feet are as important as our hands for our survival and success as a species. We tend to take them for granted, yet the many millions of modern humans who run either competitively or for recreation, or who play sports such as soccer, tennis, and badminton, or who ride, or dance, or swim, or climb, or who stand and walk as part of their work, all depend on their feet. We submit them to unreasonable loads, and expect them to survive our pounding them on hard pavements. We also add insult to injury by squeezing them into fashionable but uncomfortable footwear which does not conform to the shape of the foot.

All this means that many professionals make their living caring for our feet. Worldwide many hundreds of thousands of professional people spend most of their working life looking after the foot. They include orthopaedic surgeons, rheumatologists, diabetologists, orthotists and prosthetists, physical therapists, and podiatrists of whom there are at least 15,000 in the United States of America alone.

In the English language there are two classic books about the foot, both by anatomists. In 1935 the American anatomist Dudley Morton wrote the first edition of *The Human Foot*, and in Great Britain Frederick Wood Jones' seminal book, *Structure and Function as Seen in the Foot*, was published in 1944. But since these pioneering efforts great strides have been made in our understanding of the evolution and function of the foot. This book is not intended as a replacement for the Morton and Wood Jones monographs, but instead it is designed to provide contemporary users and healers of the foot with some context about feet. Neither is it intended to be a clinical textbook. Instead, we hope it will appeal to a wide constituency, including the professionals who care for feet, and to the many categories of `users', such as long distance runners and soccer and tennis players who depend on their feet to take them where they want to be, whether it is the finishing line of a marathon, or a place on a field or a court from where they can kick the winning goal, or play the decisive shot.

This book, the combined effort of an orthopaedic surgeon and an anatomist/palaeoanthropologist, is not intended to be comprehensive but to stimulate readers to go off on their own voyages of discovery. We have subtitled it *A Companion to Clinical Studies* because we hope that clinicians will find within its covers information that will deepen their understanding of the function and evolutionary history of this intriguing structure.

Writing any book always requires help from others. LK thanks the many friends and former colleagues who provided assistance. These include David Bowsher, Director of Research at the Pain Relief Foundation, Liverpool; Professor Robin Crompton of The University of Liverpool; Professor Adrian Lees of Liverpool John

Moore's University; Professor Phillip Tobias at his alma mater, The University of the Witwatersrand, Johannesburg; Susan Barnett, senior research fellow of The University of the West of England and member of the Foot Pressure Interest Group; Peter Seitz of Novel Gmbh, Munich; and Roger Mann, Oakland, California. All were invaluable sources of information and advice. In addition, John Kirkup, a retired orthopaedic surgeon in Bath, was LK's advisor on history, and Drs. Harish Nirula and Harry Brown of the Artificial Limb Fitting Centre at the Wrexham Maelor Hospital gave generously of their time and expertise to provide information about amputations and prostheses. Alun Jones and Andrew Biggs of the Photographic Department at the Robert Jones and Agnes Hunt Orthopaedic Hospital, Oswestry were a bastion of support and dealt efficiently with all the illustrations. My secretary Anne Leatham cheerfully coped with the long hours involved in typing draft chapters and references. Last, but not least, I am grateful for the support and constructive criticism which were always available from my wife, Naomi, and from my younger son, Paul.

BW is particularly grateful to four of his teachers. Eldred Walls taught him the anatomy of the foot, Michael Day introduced him to palaeoanthropology, Owen Lewis emphasised the importance of rigorous comparative anatomy, and Leslie Klenerman taught him orthopaedics. BW and NG are also especially grateful to Brian Richmond and Elizabeth Strasser who reviewed drafts of Chapter 1; any errors that remain are due to our intransigence. We appreciate help from Phillip Williams and Matt Skinner for generating figures and tables for Chapters 1 and 2. We thank Pilou Bazin for providing translations of articles in French. We are also grateful to the many experts, especially Osbjorn Pearson, Jennifer Clack, Will Harcourt-Smith, and Susan C. Antón, who patiently answered our questions and enquiries, as well as to the authors and publishers who allowed us to include their illustrations in this volume. BW thanks the Henry Luce Foundation for support and NG wishes to acknowledge the support of an NSF IGERT Graduate Studentship Award.

Leslie Klenerman, Bernard Wood

Contents

1
Early Evolution of the Foot

The history of life can be best understood using the analogy of a tree. All living things, be they animals, plants, fungi, bacteria, or viruses are on the outside of the tree, but they are all descended from a common ancestor at its base. The evolutionary history of all these living forms is represented by the branches within the tree. Modern humans are at the end of a relatively short twig. There is reliable genetic evidence to suggest that our nearest neighbor on the Tree of Life is the chimpanzee, with another African ape, the gorilla, being the next closest neighbour. The combined chimp/human twig is part of a small higher primate branch, which is part of a larger primate branch, which is just a small component of the bough of the Tree of Life that includes all animals (Figure 1.1).

This chapter looks into the branches of the Tree of Life to reconstruct the 'deep' evolutionary history of modern human feet. Our feet are unique. No other living animal has feet like ours, but as we show in the next chapter some of our extinct ancestors and cousins had feet that were like those of modern humans. What type of animals showed the first signs of appendages that eventually gave rise to primate feet? What can we tell about these distant ancestors and cousins that will help us make sense of the more recent evolutionary history of modern human feet? We trace the emergence of simple, primitive, paired limbs and then examine how selective forces have resulted in the various types of foot structures we see in some of the major groups of living mammals. Our focus then narrows to the early evolutionary history of the Primate order so that in the next chapter we can concentrate on the more recent evolutionary history of the human foot.

From Fins to Feet

The first animals to develop appendages, the precursors of primitive limbs of land vertebrates, lived in seas, lakes, and rivers. The pioneers of land were called tetrapods and they may have ventured out of water as early as the Upper Devonian period, approximately 370 million years ago (Mya). However, due to the paucity of fossils, palaeontologists have difficulty piecing together why tetrapods developed limbs in the first place and what caused this terrestrial radiation. There is evidence that seeking a home on land did not initially drive the growth of limbs and feet. *Acanthostega*, an early member of the lineage that includes terrestrial vertebrates, possessed fore- and hindlimbs effective for propulsion in water, but

---

Chapter co-written by Nicole L. Griffin.

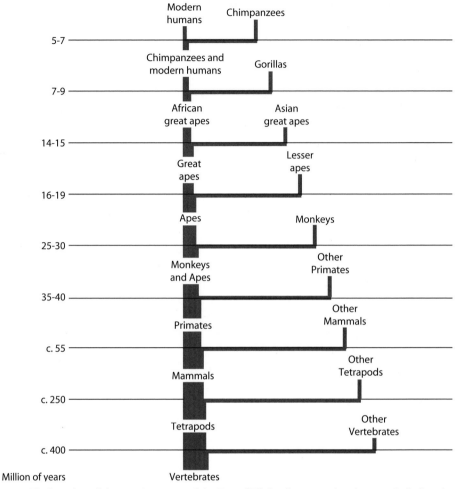

Figure 1.1. The branches of the vertebrate part of the Tree of Life leading to modern humans, including the approximate ages of the major branching points.

its wrists and ankles were not strong enough to provide support for locomotion on land [1]. Some vertebrate palaeontologists argue that the earliest tetrapods emerged in shallow swamps. This theory is supported by 365-million-year-old tetrapod trackways in Ireland [2]. Scientists believe the tetrapod who made these tracks was not walking on dry land, but was using its limbs partly as supports and partly as paddles to make its way through shallow water. They argue that if it had been walking on dry land, its tail would have left an imprint. However, it is possible *Acanthostega* is a representative of a tetrapod line that had adapted to living on the land and returned to the water. Some researchers think that a creature contemporaneous with *Acanthostega* named *Hynerpeton*, which has a forelimb strong enough to support it on dry land, may have been the one of the first tetrapods [2].

One reason put forward to explain the adaptive radiation of tetrapods is that they moved onto the land during unusually dry spells. If a water hole was drying up it made sense to venture onto the land to find a different, more reliable source of water [3,4]. However, the behaviour of the modern lungfish argues against this explanation, for when there is a drought it simply buries itself in the mud. This prevents desiccation, and allows it to survive until wetter conditions prevail. The 'water seeking' hypothesis is also weakened by the existence of aquatic creatures that can move across the land without possessing limbs. Eels, for example, which have only very abbreviated fins, make substantial excursions onto the land during the spawning season. Indeed, digitlike appendages are not exclusive to terrestrial vertebrates, for they are found in the Sargassum frogfish (Figure 1.2), an obligate aquatic dweller [1].

Currently, palaeontologists are more inclined to favour a scenario where either, or both, resource availability and predation were the driving forces behind the evolution of limbed tetrapods. It is possible that during the Upper Devonian the combination of an increase in aquatic predators and resource competition forced tetrapods to venture onto the land where their vulnerable larvae or juvenile offspring would be safer, and where food, in the form of arthropods, was more plentiful [1,5].

For the tetrapod, life on land required a change in both the respiratory system and the appendages. The replacement of gills with lungs allowed land-dwellers to inhale air and exchange oxygen for carbon dioxide. A nonaquatic environment exposed tetrapods to gravitational forces, and the development of fore- and hindlimbs lifted the thorax off the ground [6]. Not only did paired limbs replace paired fins, but also the relationship between the pectoral and pelvic girdles changed dramatically. Like their osteichthyan (bony vertebrate) ancestors, most liv-

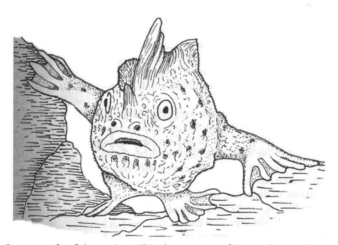

Figure 1.2. The Sargassum frogfish remains still in the presence of its prey by grasping vegetation with its digit-like appendages. (Reprinted with permission from Clack JE. *Gaining Ground: he Origin and Early Evolution of Tetrapods,* page 103, Indiana University Press 2002.)

ing bony fish have pectoral fins that are larger than their pelvic fins [1]. However, when the tetrapods shifted to the land in most cases their pectoral limbs, or fore-limbs, became smaller than their pelvic, hindlimb, counterparts [1,5]. In addition, with the establishment of a direct connection between the hindlimb and the ver-tebral column [5–7] and the fusion of the os coxa [5], the tetrapod pelvic girdle became a stable and powerful lever for transferring force from the hindlimb to the axial skeleton. Also, unlike in living fish in which each half of the pelvic girdle is anchored independently to the body wall, both halves of the tetrapod pelvic girdle meet in the midline to form a pubic symphysis, therefore providing more structural support. Other characteristics of the hindlimb unique to tetrapods include a deeper socket where the femoral head articulates with the pelvic girdle to create a more stable joint [1,8]. In addition, the lowermost vertebrae unite with the equivalent ribs to form a wide sacrum onto which leg and tail muscles insert [1,8].

The proximal regions of both the forelimbs and hindlimbs of tetrapods retain the skeletal formulae seen in the pectoral and pelvic fins, respectively, of bony fish [1]. In the tetrapod, the proximal segment (stylopodium) of the forelimb and hindlimb consists of the humerus and femur, respectively. The distal segment (zeugopodium) consists of the radius and ulna in the forelimb, and the tibia and fibula in the hindlimb. However, it is at the distal ends of the limbs where the dis-tinctiveness of tetrapods is evident. In humans and most other tetrapods, the autopodium consists of carpals, metacarpals, and phalanges in the forelimb and tarsals, metatarsals, and phalanges in the hindlimb. Very few lobe-finned fish (the closest fish relatives to tetrapods) possess homologues to tetrapod metacarpals and metatarsals and respective phalanges [1,9–11]. Although the standard num-ber of digits in contemporary tetrapods is five, with exceptions being birds who commonly have four toes and horses who have one toe, investigators are unsure why pentadactyly is the most widespread digital formula in living tetrapods and how many times it evolved (Figure 1.3). Pentadactly may have not been the prim-itive condition because the early tetrapod, *Ichthyostega*, had seven digits [1].

The standard early tetrapod pentadactyl hindlimb was arranged in three rows (Figure 1.4). The proximal row consisted of the tibiale, the intermedium, and the fibu-lare. The middle row consisted of four centrales [12]. The distal row comprised five tarsals and a prehallux along with their respective metatarsals and phalanges [12,13].

Foot Diversity

About 90 million years after the appearance of the first primitive tetrapods, around 310 Mya, the earliest members of the reptilian lineage were the first ani-mals to lay eggs on land. The morphology of these early reptiles suggests they were more committed to a terrestrial life style than either their amphibian ancestors or modern-day amphibians. The propulsive thrust of the hindlimb

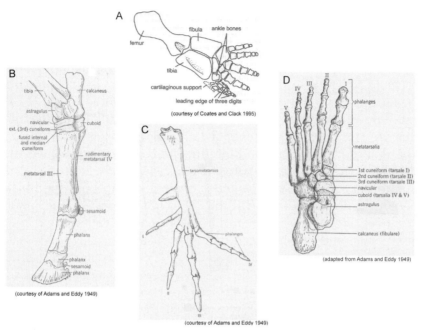

Figure 1.3. Pedal digit number varies among extinct and living tetrapods. *Ichthyostega* possessed seven digits (A). (Coates, M.I. and Clack, J.A. 1995. Romer's Gap - tetrapod origins and terrestriality. In Arsenault, M., Lelivre, H. & Janvier, P., (Eds) Proceedings of the 7th International Symposium on Early Vertebrates. Bulletin du Muséum national d'Histoire naturelle, Paris, pp. 373-388. © Publications Scientifiques du Muséum national d'Histoire naturelle, Paris.) While contemporary horses have one digit (B), chickens have four digits (C), and modern humans have five digits (D). (Reprinted with permission from Adams and Eddy [102, pp. 235–238].)

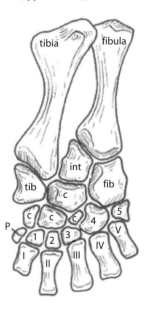

Figure 1.4. The lower limb of an early tetrapod, *Trematops milleri*. tib, tibiale; int, intermedium; fib, fibulare; c, centrale; p, prehallux; 1-5, tarsals; I-V, metatarsals. (Reproduced with permission from Lewis OJ. The Homologies of the Mammalian Tarsal Bones. J Anat. 1964;98:195-208. Blackwell Publishing Ltd.)

was improved by increasing the scope for muscle attachment on the sacrum. In addition, modifications to the foot allowed a more rapid locomotion in reptiles compared to their predecessors [6]. During the early evolution of the reptiles, the number of centralia became reduced [12]. Having already appeared in some of their primitive tetrapod ancestors, the reptilian calcaneum and talus (also called the astragalus) were recognizable entities. It is accepted that the calcaneum developed from an elongated fibulare [12,14], but the origin(s) of the talus are still debated. Gegenbaur [15] suggested the talus was formed from the union of the tibiale and intermedium, and others argued that the intermedium is the sole precursor to the talus [12,16–19]. Steiner [20] made a third suggestion, that the two centrales coalesced with both the tibiale and intermedium to form the talus. On the other hand, Berman and Henrici [21] have identified a fossil talus showing sutural lines demarcating where the intermedium, tibiale, and proximal centrale have fused. This supports Peabody's [22] hypothesis that the talus was formed by the union of these bones.

It was not until the Triassic Period (~230 Mya) that limbs began to be situated beneath the body. This change, which improved bodily support and made locomotion more efficient, is especially evident in the postcranial morphology of bipedal archosaurs, one group of the Triassic reptiles (Figure 1.5). Because their forelimbs were no longer involved in supporting the body, their forelimbs and

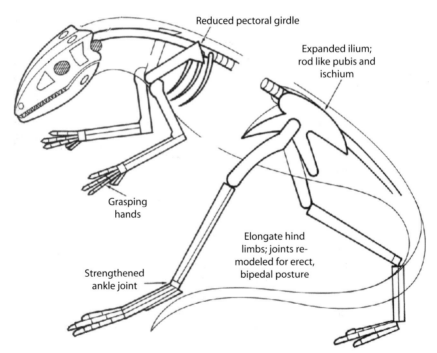

Reduced pectoral girdle

Expanded ilium; rod like pubis and ischium

Grasping hands

Elongate hind limbs; joints re-modeled for erect, bipedal posture

Strengthened ankle joint

Figure 1.5. The body plan of a bipedal archosaur. (Reprinted with permission from Radinsky L, *The Evolution of the Vertebrate Design, page 109,* Chicago: University of Chicago Press 1987.)

forelimb girdle became more gracile, and the pelvic girdle became more robust and expanded its contact with the vertebral column. This helped to transmit body weight and increased the area available for the attachment of the muscles involved in locomotion. The hindlimbs were also lengthened, and were brought closer to the midline. A hinge joint was established where the talus and calcaneum meet with the fibula and tibia. This would have improved the transmission of body weight and increased the potential for fore–aft motion of the hindlimb, thus saving energy and increasing speed of locomotion. Bipedal archosaurs probably walked on their digits; their tarsals did not come in contact with the ground [6].

Pterosaurs evolved from archosaurs and, as their name suggests, they were specialised for flight. Their forelimbs were transformed into wings, and their hindlimbs retained the form of their archosaur relatives. The ancestry of modern birds can also be traced back to the archosaurs. Living birds stand upright, with most of their weight in front of the attachment of the hindlimbs. The femur and tibia are oriented so that the joint between them more or less forms a right angle. This prevents birds from falling forward [23,24]. Birds stand on their toes, with three digits pointing forwards and one back. Their metatarsals are elongated and are fused with the tarsal bones. This combined elongated tarsometatarsus forming a simple hinge joint enabled birds to take longer strides [14,23].

Whereas some archosaurs became bipedal and/or were specialised for flight, others turned to an aquatic life (Figure 1.6). The appendages of these marine reptiles were customised into paddles. One group, the plesiosaurs, maintained a

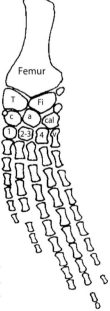

Figure 1.6. The paddlelike hindlimb of *Plesiosaurus* increases the number of phalanges in each ray. T, tibia; Fi, fibula; c, centrale; a, astragalus; cal, calcaneus; 1-V, tarsals. (From Carroll RL. Patterns and Processes of Vertebrate Evolution, page 252, 1997. Reprinted with the permission of Cambridge University Press.)

five-digit autopodium and added several more tarsals and phalanges [24]. Marine reptiles, such as icthyosaurs, also increased the number of their foot phalanges, but reduced their autopodium to three digits. These creatures became so specialised for life in water that it is probable they were incapable of venturing beyond the shoreline [6].

Mammals evolved about 225 Mya from a group called the therapsids, or mammallike reptiles. In mammals, the navicular is recognizable, but the fifth primitive tarsal bone is lost. The origins of the navicular and the fate of the fifth tarsal are contested. Schaeffer [25] and Romer [26] argued the navicular is a homologue of one of the centrales, but Steiner [20] suggested the navicular was formed from the amalgamation of two centrales. The majority of studies suggest that the therapsid navicular was formed from the union of the tibiale and centrale [12,16,17,27–30]. In primitive mammals, only four tarsals, the three cuneiforms and the cuboid, articulate with the metatarsals. Steiner [20] acknowledged the fifth tarsal as lost and identified the fourth as the cuboid. In contrast, Lewis [12] suggested that the cuboid is formed from the fusion of the fourth and fifth tarsals.

With the emergence of mammals, changes to limb morphology led to even more types of locomotor repertoires. The most revolutionary of these morphological changes were the superimposition of the talus over the calcaneum and the elimination of the articulation between the fibula and calcaneum. Thus, the weight-bearing function of the fibula was reduced [31,32]. Other changes in the hindlimb morphology included moving the feet even closer to the body and knees that point forward. At the hip and ankle joints the elongation of two bony processes, the greater trochanter of the femur at the hip, and the posteriorly-projecting calcaneum at the ankle (the Achilles heel), increased the mechanical efficiency of muscles. The greater trochanter of the femur improved the moment arm of the gluteal muscles, and at the ankle the elongated calcaneum improved the moment arm of the muscles attached to the Achilles tendon [6].

The main bony elements of the hindlimb, the stylopodium and zeugopodium, are relatively conservative and have retained their primitive morphology throughout most of the evolutionary history of the tetrapods. In contrast, the autopodium at the distal extremity of the hindlimb has become highly specialised, especially within mammals. As outlined by Hildebrand [33], we recognize and introduce five locomotor groups. These are not grouped according to phylogenetic criteria, but according to shared mechanical demands. First are runners and jumpers; second, diggers and crawlers; third, climbers; fourth, swimmers and divers; and fifth, fliers and gliders.

Members of the fast-running mammalian group include ungulates, and hopping rodents and marsupials. Among the ungulates, the even-toed artiodactyls, such as deer, sheep, and elk, have evolved a foot skeleton that comprises only the third and fourth metatarsals, also called metapodials, that are fused together to form the cannon bone. The phalanges associated with those metatarsals are each encased in a hoof. The other main ungulate group, the odd-toed perissodactyls, which includes horses, have just a single metapodial, and their phalanges are encased in one hoof. The cannon bone and the single metapodial provide sufficient strength, and their light weight allows their owners to run quickly [6].

The distal segments of the hindlimb in hopping mammals are differently adapted for speed. The length of the hindlimb is proportional to the distance of muscular force used during jumping. In turn, this distance directly correlates to the height and distance of the jump. To lengthen the hindlimb, some mammals, such as rodents, kangaroos, and primates have elongated their ankle bones [6].

Members of the digging and crawling group have reduced their forelimbs and hindlimbs so that they do not obstruct movement through narrow burrows. Some burrowers such as the tuco-tuco rodent use their forefeet and hindfeet to push dirt out of the way. The foot pads of these creatures have been widened for more effective use [33].

The third group consists of climbers. For most, the feet have been modified to grip the substrate. For example, opposums and most primates have divergent first toes. As a secondarily-adapted climber, the Central American porcupine is able to fold together the medial and lateral sides of its foot to grasp a tree limb. Another approach to grasping is exhibited by the anteater. This creature opposes its heel to make contact with its two toes. Primates, anteaters, and porcupines have pads on their hands and feet for cushioning and to create friction during climbing. Some climbers, such as squirrels, have claws that also aid in adhering to the support [33].

Swimmers and divers, such as whales and dolphins, have evolved streamlined bodies and short limbs. Mammals that lead both a terrestrial and aquatic life, such as sea lions and seals, have converted their fore- and hindfeet into paddles by lengthening their digits and developing webbing between them [6].

The only mammals who became specialised for flight are bats. Their forelimb bones, especially their lateral digits, have become elongated as struts for wings, whereas their hips and ankle joints and their hooklike digits are adapted for hanging upside down [6].

Modern humans are the only living primate, indeed they are the only living mammal, that is an obligatory striding biped. Obligatory bipeds are animals that as adults rely solely on their hindlimbs for support and propulsion when walking on the ground. It is almost certain that this very special type of primate locomotion evolved within the last five to eight million years. The rest of this chapter and the next trace the evolutionary history of modern human bipedal locomotion.

Modern humans belong to the order Primates, the suborder Anthropoidea, the superfamily Hominoidea, the family Hominidae, the tribe Hominini, and the genus *Homo* (Figure 1.7). A more reader-friendly way to express this very technical description is that modern humans are one of the apes, that apes are in turn part of the monkey and ape subgroup of the primates, and that this primate subgroup originated in the distant past, at least 60 million years ago, from the common ancestor of all living and fossil primates. Thus, if we are to understand the evolutionary context

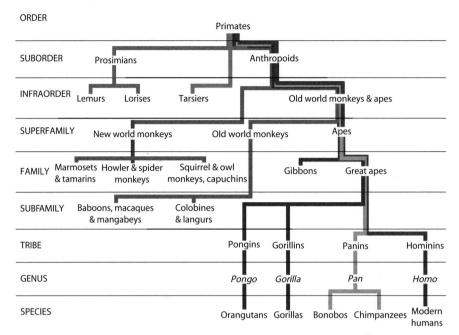

ORDER
Primates

SUBORDER   Prosimians   Anthropoids

INFRAORDER   Lemurs   Lorises   Tarsiers   Old world monkeys & apes

SUPERFAMILY   New world monkeys   Old world monkeys   Apes

FAMILY   Marmosets Howler & spider   Squirrel & owl   Gibbons   Great apes
         & tamarins   monkeys   monkeys, capuchins

SUBFAMILY   Baboons, macaques   Colobines
             & mangabeys   & langurs

TRIBE   Pongins   Gorillins   Panins   Hominins

GENUS   Pongo   Gorilla   Pan   Homo

SPECIES   Orangutans Gorillas   Bonobos Chimpanzees Modern
                                                                            humans

Figure 1.7. Primate taxonomy.

of the modern human foot we need to find out what information comparative anatomy and the fossil record can tell us about a series of common ancestors. These are, in order from oldest to youngest, the common ancestor of all primates, the common ancestor of anthropoid primates (monkeys and apes), the common ancestor of apes, the common ancestor of the African apes including modern humans, and finally the common ancestor of modern humans and chimpanzees. Only then will we be in a position to try to make sense of the human fossil record to see what sort of feet our cousins and immediate ancestors had.

Primate Feet

Before discussing the evolutionary history of the primate foot, we first review the feet of living primates so we can better understand how they relate to differences in primate locomotion. This survey of the way living primates have modified the design of the primitive mammalian foot provides a background for our review of the fossil primates ancestral to chimpanzees and modern humans.

All primates, except the loris, have five functional digits. Almost all the feet of living primates, with the conspicuous exception of modern humans, have a divergent big toe or hallux [32]. This is an adaptation for grasping. The thumblike 'saddle' joint between the hallux and the medial cuneiform combined with the contractions of the toe flexors allow the big toe to meet with the lateral toes in a grasping position. Movements between the talus and the navicular, and the calcaneum and cuboid, allow inversion and eversion movements that help to turn the foot into an efficient grasping organ [34].

The design of the feet of living primates is governed by posture (while resting and eating) as well as by locomotion. Researchers unite locomotion and posture and call the two 'positional behaviour' [35]. However, the categories we review below refer in the main to locomotion, although inevitably locomotion and posture are interrelated. It is worth noting that unlike modern humans, all other primates have a locomotor repertoire that includes various kinds of locomotion and their feet reflect this compromise.

Vertical Clinging and Leaping

Some primates adopt vertical clinging as their posture at rest and then use leaping in order to move between vertical supports (Figure 1.8). As an adaptation to clinging, indriids have evolved a unique gripping mechanism (Figure 1.9). There

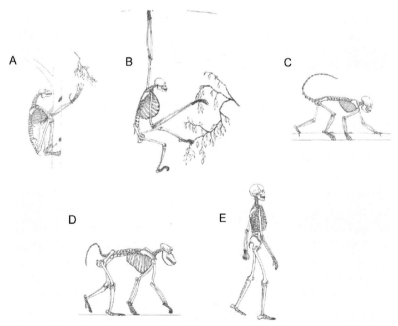

Figure 1.8. Four positional behaviours found in the Primate order (A) vertical clinging and leaping, (B) suspension, (C) arboreal quadrupedalism, (D) terrestrial quadrupedalism, (E) bipedalism. (Reprinted from Primate Adaptation and Evolution, 2nd ed., Fleagle JG, 298-303, Copyright (1999), with permission from Elsevier. Illustrations by Stephen Nash.)

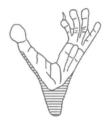

Figure 1.9. The 'cleft' in the indriid foot allows for a wide and secure grip during climbing. (Reprinted from Gebo D. *Postcranial Adaptations in Nonhuman primates*, pages 175–198, Northern Illinois University Press 1993.)

is a deep cleft between the big toe and the second toe, and the flexor muscles have increased in size [34]. Adaptations for leaping include a long hindlimb built for power at take-off and shock absorption during landing. In tarsiers, superficial flexor muscles are employed for propulsion. Although the tarsal region of the foot varies among leapers, most have an elongated calcaneum and navicular to increase the load arm [35]. Other characteristics common in primates who leap include a large expanded facet on the talus for the fibula in order to increase mobility, and the presence of squatting facets located where the talar body and neck meet. These latter facets suggest that the foot is bent up against the leg (i.e., dorsiflexion) during clinging and prior to leaping [31]. Dorsiflexion and plantarflexion of the foot are promoted by the fusion of the fibula and tibia at the ankle joint in some taxa [35].

Suspension

Suspensory primates hang below tree branches using a combination of arm and leg supports (Figure 1.8). The feet of suspensory primates are similar to their hands. The big toe, like the thumb, is well developed and the toe phalanges are long and curved for grasping branches. Sometimes specialised suspensory primates use their feet to grasp a support so that they can use both hands to feed. The long phalanges of the lateral toes hook above the support and the big toe hangs freely or curls around larger branches. Lorises also have a well-developed hallux and strong flexor or toe-curling muscles. Long toes coupled with a wide range of movement at their tarsal joints provide the agility needed to adjust to a variety of supports [34]. The tarsal bones of loris feet have become realigned so that the medially projecting big toe can grasp quite large tree trunks [34,36]. Other modifications of the foot of a suspensory primate include a wide range of movement at the ankle joint, a short calcaneum, and modifications to the short muscles that flex the toes to increase grasping power. Unlike the feet of arboreal clinging and leaping primates, or the feet of terrestrial primates, the feet of suspensory primates are especially mobile [35].

Quadrupedalism

The least specialised of the four basic locomotor patterns of primates is quadrupedalism. This form of locomotion uses all four limbs to carry the weight of the body. Primate quadrupedalism can be divided into two categories, arboreal quadrupedalism and terrestrial quadrupedalism. In arboreal quadrupedal primates (Figure 1.8), the foot structure is adapted for grasping, but not to the extent it is in vertical climbers. Asymmetry of the tibio-talar facet allows the foot to be inverted while the toes are used for grasping [35]. Terrestrial quadrupedal primates (Figure 1.8) have robust tarsals and metatarsals. The toes are relatively short and joint mobility is limited. Terrestrial quadrupeds also have a reduced hallux compared to most arboreal quadrupeds because there is less need for grasping [37]. The feet of knuckle-walkers (chimpanzees and gorillas) exhibit a mosaic of features characteristic of terrestrial and arboreal quadrupedalism as well as climbing. During knuckle-walking (Figure 1.10), the body weight is transferred through the foot via the long, broad, low transverse arch to the distal metatarsals. The first metatarsal is designed to serve two functions. It acts as a lever during push-off on the ground, and as a vise while moving through the trees [38].

Although both the forelimb and hindlimb are employed in primate quadrupedal locomotion, there tends to be more emphasis on the hindlimb [39]. Contrary to most other quadrupedal placental mammals who locomote using a 'lateral' gait sequence, the majority of primate quadrupeds use a 'diagonal' sequence [40]. When describing the order in which the four limbs make contact with the substrate, it is conventional to start the gait sequence at the

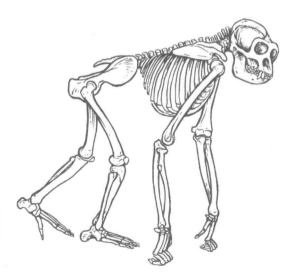

Figure 1.10. Knuckle-walking gorilla. (Reprinted from Primate Adaptation and Evolution, 2nd ed., Fleagle JG, 247, Copyright (1999), with permission from Elsevier. Illustration by Stephen Nash.)

point when the right hindlimb is set down on the substrate. In a 'diagonal' quadrupedal gait, the next limb to touch the substrate is the left forelimb, then the left hindlimb, and the last limb to contact the substrate is the right forelimb.

Bipedalism

The only form of primate locomotion that depends solely on the hindlimbs for locomotion is bipedalism (Figure 1.8). The upper limbs and trunk are involved in bipedalism, but they are used for balance and modulation, not locomotion as such. Modern humans are the only living primates that are habitual bipeds. Most primates use bipedalism infrequently (e.g., gibbons and chimpanzees) and a few specialised leapers hop bipedally when on the ground. In contrast to primate quadrupeds, the centre of gravity at rest in a biped is between the feet. The centre of gravity, however, moves forward when one leg moves forward carrying the body with it [41]. A simple 'walking cycle' (i.e., the sequence of events between the times the right heel meets the ground) is divided into the stance phase (i.e., when that foot is on the ground) and the swing phase (i.e., when that foot is off the gound). For 80% of the cycle one or the other hindlimb is in the swing phase and for 20% of the cycle both feet are on the ground. During running the feet do not touch the ground at the same time. With this background, we discuss bipedal striding as it specifically relates to muscle contraction at key joints of the lower limb. At heel strike (the beginning of a walking cycle) flexion has occurred at the hip, the knee is extended, and the leg is laterally rotated. Body weight is moved over the supporting limb by the action of the adductors of the leg in the stance phase. Just before toe-off, body weight is transferred to the hallux. At this point of the stance phase, the hip and the knee are extended. The stance phase is now completed. The swing phase begins with flexion at the hip and knee. The knee then extends when the leg in the swing phase passes the supporting leg. The leg in the swing phase laterally rotates as it prepares for heel strike [42].

To convert the foot from a grasping, handlike appendage to a rigid lever suitable for a bipedal gait, it was necessary to have both a lever arm, the calcaneal tuberosity, and a load arm, in this case a stable tarsus and an adducted robust hallux. Inasmuch as toes were not needed for grasping, they were shortened. The neck of the talus became less obliquely oriented than in quadrupedal primates so that it was aligned with the long axis of the foot. Strong ligaments on the plantar surface bind the tarsals and metatarsals together and function as shock absorbers when the foot takes the weight of the body during the stance phase. A longitudinal arch made of bones and ligaments allows body weight to be transferred from the hindfoot to the forefoot via the lateral side of the foot [42,43].

Pads, Claws and Nails

A review of the main types of living foot structures would not be complete without some mention of the superficial soft tissues of the foot. These include the hairless skin pads that protect the underside of the foot and the claws and nails that function as specialised extensions of the foot. In his survey of mammalian feet, Whipple [44] noted there are cutaneous pads on the plantar surface of the foot, one at the tips of each digit and six proximal pads. Four of the six pads are at the junctions of the phalanges and metatarsals. The remaining two, the thenar and hypothenar pads, are located at the medial and lateral aspects of the ankle, respectively. Lorises retain all six of the proximal pads on the foot, and mouse lemurs have done the same, but with the addition of an accessory pad on their first rays (Figure 1.11). Living apes and modern humans have also retained all six proximal pads, but they are only distinguished as clear entities in fetal feet [45]. Later in development they tend to merge and the hairless skin of the pads is covered with fine, whorllike ridges only at the fingertips. These cutaneous pads have two main functional roles. Specialised sensory receptors on the ridges provide increased sensitivity to touch, and the ridges together with the sweat glands help provide friction when the foot is used to grip arboreal supports. In prosimian feet, these specialised epidermal ridges are only found on the apical pads, but in the anthropoids, including humans, the ridges are more widely distributed on the sole of the foot. Cartmill [46] has linked this difference to allometry. In primates, the coalescence of pads scales with body size.

The 'skin' that surrounds the distal pedal phalanges of mammals is variable in both form and function. Its form includes the massive claws of large-bodied carnivores, the hooves of horses, and the delicate flat nails of primates (Figure 1.12). This relationship between structure and function is very evident when

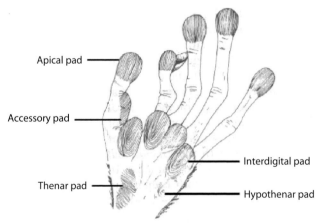

Figure 1.11. The foot of the mouse lemur (*Microcebus murinus*) includes an accessory pad on the hallux, a specialization seen in some primates. Note the grooming claw on the second digit. (Martin, Robert D. *Primate Origins and Evolution*. © R.D. Martin. Reprinted by permission of Princeton University Press.)

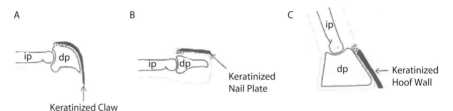

Figure 1.12. The morpology of the mammalian claw (A), nail (B), and hoof (C). ip, intermediate phalanx; dp, distal phalanx. (Reprinted from Hamrick MW. Development and evolution of the mammalian limb: adaptive diversification of nails, hooves, and claws. Evol Dev. 2001;3(5):355–63.)

one considers the role of claws and nails in primates. For example, marmosets use their secondarily-derived claws on their hands and feet to grip a tree trunk when they extract gum [47]. This type of feeding specialisation would be impossible if these primates had flat nails. However, despite specialisations such as those seen in marmosets, all primates have a nail on the big toe. In some prosimians, one or more pedal digits bear clawlike nails specialised for grooming fur. Compared to regular claws, 'toilet claws' are longer, more curved, and less sharp (Figure 1.11).

Ancient Primates

Functional interpretations of the feet of our distant human ancestors are based on analogies with similar looking feet of living primates and by using morphology to predict the functional demands placed on the feet. This final section traces the evolution of the primate foot during the Paleocene (65–55 Mya), Eocene (55–35 Mya), Oligocene (35–25 Mya), and Miocene (25–5 Mya). Because our focus is on the evolution of the human foot, fossil platyrrhines (New World Monkeys) are not discussed for they diverged from the catarrhines (Old World Monkeys and apes, including humans) approximately 30 to 35 Mya.

Little is known about the locomotion of the immediate mammalian ancestors of the primates, but it is most likely that these mouse to rat-sized creatures were at least partly arboreal [48]. Their feet were capable of inversion and eversion and their phalanges look as if they had narrow pointed claws and powerful flexor muscles [31]. The grasping foot is likely to have been the primitive condition for primates, for Steiner [49] noted that during the early stages of mammalian development *in utero*, the elongation of the medial cuneiform moves the first ray medially so that there is a gap between it and the lateral rays.

The first primates appear to have been small nocturnal animals with grasping hands and feet, nails, and a diagonal sequence gait adapted for movement on thin, flexible branches [50,51]. Some suggest that the first primates were Plesiadapiformes (Figure 1.13), which lived during the Paleocene epoch [52]. Although many researchers recognise that Plesiadapiformes share some morpho-

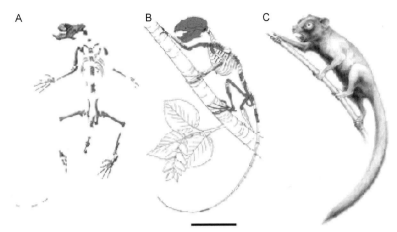

Figure 1.13. The plesiadapiform, *Carpolestes simpsoni* (56 Mya) possessed an abducted nail-bearing big toe capable of opposition, and an ankle designed for leaping. Although Bloch and Boyer [52] suggest these traits as well as others link Carpolestes to Euprimates, Kirk et al. (2003) [104] warn that a clawless opposable hallux is also found in living rodents and marsupials. (Reprinted with permission from Bloch JI, Boyer DM. Grasping primate origins. Science. 2002;298(5598):1606–10. Copyright 2002 AAAS.)

logical traits exclusively with primates [43,53], Plesiadapiformes have unique specialisations that may preclude them from being ancestral to primates [35].

Several key features of the plesiadapiform foot include a talus resting directly on the calcaneum in such a manner as to allow the calcaneum to protract and retract during inversion and eversion of the foot. Researchers also include a well-developed calcaneonavicular ligament and flexor digitorum fibularis, a distinguishable talar head and neck, a small or absent talar canal, a subtalar axis occupying an oblique position relative to the long axis of the foot [54], and an opposable hallux bearing a nail [52] as plesiadapiform characters.

The Eocene epoch sees the first evidence of Euprimates, a radiation of creatures that are undeniably primates. Eocene Euprimates belong to two families, the Adapidae and the Omomyidae. Fossil adapids and omomyids show several novel features of the foot not found in the feet of the Plesiadapiformes, but they are found in the feet of modern-day prosimian primates that are vertical clingers and leapers [31,55]. These include adaptations of the calcaneum and calcaneal joints to increase the range of rotation of the midtarsal region and the speed of plantarflexion [31].

By the time of the Oligocene epoch (37–25 Mya) researchers are confident they can recognise the postoanial remains early relatives of living anthropoids (monkeys, apes, including humans) in the fossil record [35,53,56]. Two main families of primates are present during this epoch, the Parapithecidae and the Propliopithecidae. The foot of one parapithecid, *Apidium phiomense*, shares adaptations with the feet of terrestrial anthropoids in that it displays evidence of reduced mobility of the subtalar and transverse tarsal joints and a short calcaneum. However, there are morphological features of *Apidium phiomense* that are also similar to those of living prosimians. The long lower limb and the shape of the upper ankle joint suggest *Apidium phiomense* was adapted for leaping [57].

Several researchers suggest that a lineage of Propliopithecidae includes the direct ancestors of extant catarrhines (Old World monkeys and apes, including humans) [58–61]. Foot bones, especially the calcaneum, belonging to *Aegyptopithecus zeuxis* and *Propliopithecus chirobates* indicate that these two propliopithecids were arborealists. A plantar tubercle on the calcaneum [62] and a calcaneocuboid joint designed for wide rotational capabilities suggest that their feet were designed for suspension and climbing [57]. Curvature of the medial talar trochlear rim provided extensive mobility in the foot of *Aegyptopithecus zeuxis*. The big toe was abducted, the metatarsals and phalanges were long, and the proximal phalanges curved [57]. Although *Aegyptopithecus zeuxis* is not directly related to the New World monkeys, it shares some of the same morphology. For example, *Aegyptopithecus zeuxis* retained a primitive prehallux, a tarsometatarsal sesamoid of the first ray, a feature which is only found in extant primates from the New World [31].

Miocene Primates

Approximately 21 genera of 'hominoids' have been recovered from layers of strata dating to the Miocene epoch (24–5 Mya) [35]. However, debate centres around which of these fossil primates represent true hominoids and also how each one fits into the family tree of living apes [63]. A probable basal hominoid, *Proconsul* [60,64] has a foot most comparable to those of living arboreal monkeys [63, and references therein], but also shares some pedal characteristics with great apes [65,66]. *Proconsul* and living arboreal monkeys have similar talocrural joints and transverse arches [31,65]. For example, the angle formed by the subtalar axis and the long axis of the foot is similar [31]. In addition, *Proconsul* shares with arboreal monkeys a narrow forefoot and gracile lateral metatarsals and phalanges [31]. *Proconsul's* calcaneal facets [67], long hallux [66], and relatively short and robust intermediate phalanges [66] are apelike characteristics. In particular, *Proconsul* is similar to African apes in its shape and the curvature of the talar trochlea [67] and torsion of the first and second metatarsals [65]. The hallux of *Proconsul* is strong and robust, capable of powerful grasping and together with a flexible midtarsal joint and long phalanges, the foot of this fossil primate was suited for arboreal quadrupedalism and slow climbing [31,65,66,68]. A later basal hominoid *Nacholopithecus* has long forelimbs and long pedal digits that indicate it was a forelimb-dominated arborealist [69].

The European hominoid *Dryopithecus* is a possible last common ancestor of the great apes and humans. This Miocene genus has been divided into several species [70]. Pedal remains are scarce, but a few hand phalanges and a pedal phalanx, as well as other postcranial evidence suggest *Dryopithecus* was a suspensory primate [71]. In particular, the moderately curved intermediate foot phalanx has a mediolaterally broad shaft and well-developed flexor sheath ridges. The distal articular surface indicates that a large range of flexion and extension was possible at this joint.

Currently, no fossil has been confirmed as the Miocene ape ancestral to African apes and humans. Therefore, we do not know how this creature moved about. Some researchers suggest that it would have emphasised either climbing and/or suspensory behaviour [72–79], whereas others suggest that the common ancestor of African apes and humans was a terrestrial quadruped [80,81], and several researchers are advocates for the common ancestor being a knuckle-walker and climber [82–88]. Chimpanzees and gorillas are most closely related to modern humans and because they both employ knuckle-walking (chimps more so than gorillas) it is hypothesised that the common ancestor was a knuckle-walker and climber [88]. This hypothesis is supported by Richmond and Strait's [87] survey of extant hominoids, fossil hominins, and humans. In their report, fossil hominins dating to over 3.5 million years ago show key knuckle-walking wrist traits suggesting that hominins evolved from a knuckle-walking ancestor.

Gebo [89] proposed that the most distinguishing feature of the common ancestor of the African great apes and modern humans would be the ability to place the foot in a plantigrade position on the substrate (Figure 1.14). He defines a plantigrade foot as '. . . one in which the heel contacts the surface of a terrestrial or arboreal support at the end of swing phase' [89]. Gebo [89] asserts that all other primates habitually use a semiplantigrade foot posture at the end of the swing phase, although several researchers disagree with him because they have observed New World and other Old World primates using a plantigrade foot position [90,91]. In a semiplantigrade posture, the calcaneum is lifted above the substrate and does not bear any body weight (Figure 1.15). Instead, body weight is borne on the plantar surface of the cuboid, lateral cuneiform, and navicular. To bring the foot into a plantigrade position, the calcaneum occupies an inverted position before contacting the substrate and it maintains this attitude even at midstance when body weight is transferred to the forefoot. The transfer of weight stabilises the forefoot, which is everted [89].

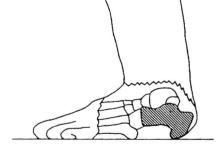

Figure 1.14. The primate foot in a plantigrade position. Only the calcaneum and fifth metatarsal make contact with the ground. (Reprinted from Gebo D. *Postcranial Adaptations in Nonhuman primates*, pages 175–198, Northern Illinois University Press 1993.)

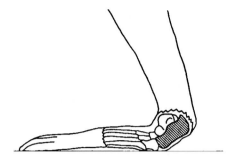

Figure 1.15. The primate foot in a semiplantigrade position. The calcaneum is lifted off the ground and the tarsals make contact with the substrate. (Reprinted from Gebo D. *Postcranial Adaptations in Nonhuman primates*, pages 175–198, Northern Illinois University Press 1993.)

Gebo [89] explains that the transition from a semiplantigrade foot to a plantigrade foot during evolution had several consequences for the feet of African great apes and humans. These include reduced subtalar mobility and morphological adjustments to the calcaneum and other tarsals. The development of a bony extension along the lateral region of the calcaneum and a prominent peroneal tubercle add stability at heel strike. Also, the calcaneum is permanently fixed in a laterally rotated position in anticipation of being inverted when the heel contacts the substrate. The cuboid is laterally rotated and lifted as is the navicular. It is suggested that the digits of the African great ape common ancestor would resemble those of chimps and gorillas in being relatively short and the big toe, although still abducted, would be less mobile [89].

The modern human and chimp lineages diverged later in the Miocene epoch. Molecular evidence suggests that this took place 5.0 to 8.0 Mya [92–94]. But, foot fossils are poorly represented in the late Miocene higher primate fossil record. Possible candidates for the modern human–chimp common ancestor (hominin–panin common ancestor) include *Sahelanthropus tchadensis* (6–7 Mya) and *Orrorin tugenensis* (5.2–5.8 Mya), but there is controversy surrounding the interpretations of the locomotor patterns of these two fossils. Brunet et al. [95] suggested that the forward location of the foramen magnum of *S. tchadensis* is consistent with it being bipedal and thus it is a hominin rather than the common ancestor of hominins and panins. But others have argued that *S. tchadensis* cannot be confidently designated a hominin because face and masticatory anatomy and the morphology of the foramen magnum are similar to those of African great apes [96].

Senut et al. [97] cite the external morphology of the neck of the femur as evidence that *O. tugenensis* was bipedal. The same authors also suggest *O. tugenensis* was a capable climber as indicated by the curved shaft of a proximal manual phalanx and the pattern of bony crests on the distal humerus. Others claim both the proximal and distal femoral anatomy lack diagnostic bipedal characteristics [98], and Haile-Selassie [99] argues that there is not yet enough evidence to decide whether *O. tugenensis* is a likely modern human–chimp common ancestor or the common ancestor of hominins. A more recent study [100] of the internal structure of an *O. tugenensis* femoral neck reveals its cortex is distinct from those of the African apes and most like the cortices of the modern human femoral necks, suggesting that it was bipedal.

Because we cannot be certain where both *S. tchadensis* and *O. tugenensis* are located with respect to the hominin twig of the Tree of Life, we must use other evidence to predict the nature of the hominin–panin common ancestor. Based on parsimony and early hominin foot morphology it would be expected that the hominin–panin ancestor would have feet more similar to chimpanzees than to modern humans. As efficient climbers, brachiators, terrestrial knuckle-walkers, and capable, but infrequent bipeds, chimpanzees possess a mosaic of pedal traits to meet these locomotor demands. Arboreal adaptations in the chimp foot include a talus with a moderately long neck and an asymmetrical trochlear surface, a calcaneocuboid joint designed for pivoting, mobile transverse tarsal joints, an abducted opposable hallux, and long and curved phalanges with prominent flexor sheath ridges [42,89]. These traits are predicted to be among those possessed by the foot of the modern human–chimp common ancestor.

Like the African ape common ancestor, the modern human–chimp common ancestor would have had a chimplike plantigrade foot. In chimps, the shape of the trochlear surface promotes medial mobility during dorsiflexion and lateral mobility during plantarflexion, therefore causing the tibia to trace an arcuate-shaped pathway as it moves over the stance phase foot. In contrast, the lateral and medial borders of the modern human trochlear surface constrain the tibia to a straighter path as it moves over the foot. The hominin–chimp common ancestor's leg would have been expected to follow the arcuate pathway, and it is unlikely to have possessed a longitudinal arch. The lack of a longitudinal arch, and the probable presence of a phenomenon called the 'midtarsal break' have implications for the gait of the modern human–chimp common ancestor (Figure 1.16. A 'midtarsal break' occurs in panins when the lateral side of the foot

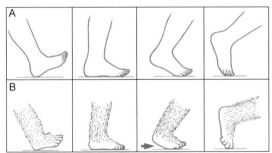

Figure 1.16. Bipedal stride in (A) a human and (B) chimpanzee. The 'midtarsal break' during the gait of the chimpanzee is noted by the arrow. (Reprinted from Aiello L, Dean C. An Introduction to Human Evolutionary Anatomy, page 508, Copyright 1990, with permission from Elsevier.)

including the calcaneum and cuboid stays in contact with the ground. As the heel is lifted off the substrate the foot pivots at the calcaneocuboid joint. It is unlikely there would have been any medial weight transfer across the forefoot of the modern human–chimp common ancestor.

In the next chapter we focus on the evolution of the foot by reviewing taxa that are almost certainly hominins. We explore the prospect that bipedalism evolved several times, and then trace how the foot of early hominins evolved into a modern humanlike foot.

References

1.   Clack J. *Gaining Ground*. Bloomington: Indiana University Press; 2002.
2.   Westenberg K. From fins to feet. *Nat Geo*. 1999; 195: 114–127.
3.   Romer A. *Man and the Vertebrates*. Chicago: Chicago University Press; 1933.
4.   Romer A. *Vertebrate Paleontology*. 2nd ed. Chicago: Chicago University Press; 1945.
5.   Young, J. *The Life of Vertebrates*. Oxford: Clarendon Press; 1981.
6.   Radinsky L. *The Evolution of the Vertebrate Design*. Chicago: University of Chicago Press; 1987.
7.   Carroll R. *Vertebrate Paleontology and Evolution*. New York: W.H. Freeman; 1988.
8.   Romer A. *Vertebrate Paleontology*. Chicago: University of Chicago Press; 1966.
9.   Ahlberg PE, Milner AR.The origin and early diversification of tetrapods. *Nature*. 1994; 368: 507–512.
10. Sordino P, Duboule D. A molecular approach to the evolution of vertebrate paired appendages. *Trends Ecol Evol*. 1996; 11: 114–119.
11. Hinchlife JR. Developmental basis of limb evolution. *Int J Dev Biol*. 2002; 46: 835–845.
12. Lewis O.J. *Functional Morphology of the Evolving Hand and Foot*. Oxford: Clarendon Press; 1989.
13. Isidro A, Gonzalez-Casanova J. A glimpse into the evolution of the hallucial tarsometatarsal joint. *Foot and Ankle Surgery*. 2002; 8: 169–174.
14. Benton M. *Vertebrate Paleontology*. Malden, MA: Blackwell; 2005.
15. Gegenbaur C. *Untersuchung zur vergleichenden Anatomie der Wirbeltiere. I. Carpus and Tarsus*. Leipzig: Englemann; 1864.
16. Baur G. Zur Morphologie des Tarsus der Säugethiere. *Morphologisches Jahrbuch*. 1884; 10: 458–461.
17. Baur G. On the morphology of the carpus and tarsus of vertebrates. *Am Nat*. 1885; 19: 718–720.
18. Romer A, Bryne F. The pes of *Diadectes*: Notes on the primitive tetrapod limb. *Palaebiologica*. 1931; 4: 25–48.
19. Romer A, Price L. Review of the Pelycosauria. *Geo Soc Am Special Paper*. 1940; 28: 538.
20. Steiner H. Die embryonale Hand-und Fussekelettentwicklung von *Tupaia*. *Verhandlungen der Schweizerischen Naturforschenden Gesellschaft*. 1951; 113: 153–154.
21. Berman D, Henrici A. Homology of the astragulus and structure and function of the tarsus of Diadectidae. *J Paleont*. 2003; 77: 172–188.
22. Peabody F. The origin of the astragalus of reptiles. *Evolution*. 1951; 5: 339–344.
23. Rogers E. *Looking at Vertebrates*. Essex: Longman; 1986.
24. Carroll R. *Patterns and Processes of Vertebrate Evolution*. Cambridge: Cambridge University Press; 1997.
25. Schaeffer B. The morphological and functional evolution of the tarsus in amphibians and reptiles. *Bull Am Mus Nat Hist*. 1941; 78: 395–472.

26. Romer A. *Vertebrate Paleontology*. Chicago: University of Chicago Press; 1955.
27. Albrecht P. Sur les homodynamies qui existent entre la main et le pied des mammiferes. *Presse medicale blege*. 1884; 36: 329–311.
28. Cope E. Fifth contribution to the knowledge of the fauna of the Permian formation of Texas and the Indian territory. *Palaeontological Bull*. 1884; 39: 28–47.
29. Cope E. The relationship between theromorphous reptiles and the monotreme. *Mammalia Proc Am Assoc Advance Sci*. 1885; 33: 471–482.
30. Bardeleben K. Ueber neue Bestandteile der Hand-und Fusswurzel der Säugethiere, sowie die normale Anlage von Rudimenten 'Überzähliger' Finger und Zehen beim Menschen. *Sitzungsberichte der jena Gesellschaft für Medizin und Naturwissen schaften*. 1885; 19: 149–164.
31. Conroy G, Rose, M. The evolution of the primate foot from the earliest primates to the Miocene hominoids. *Foot Ankle*. 1983; 3: 342–364.
32. Martin R. *Primate Origins and Evolution*. Princeton, NJ: Princeton University Press; 1990.
33. Hildebrand M. *Analysis of Vertebrate Structure*. 4th ed. New York: Wiley; 1995: 657.
34. Gebo D. Functional morphology of the foot in primates. In: Gebo D, ed. *Postcranial Adaptations in Nonhuman Primates*. DeKalb, IL: Northern Illinois University Press; 1993a:175–198.
35. Fleagle J. *Primate Adaptations and Evolution*. San Diego: Academic; 1999.
36. Gebo D. Postcranial adaptation and evolution in Lorisidae. *Primates*. 1989; 30: 347–367.
37. Strasser E. Relative development of the hallux pedal digit formulae in Cercopithecidae. *J Hum Evol*. 1994; 26:5/6: 413–440.
38. Wunderlich RE. *Pedal Form and Function in Anthropoid Primates*. In: *Doctoral Program in Anthropological Sciences*. Stony Brook: State University of New York at Stony Brook; 1999.
39. Demes AB, et al. The kinetics of primate quadrupedalism: "Hind limb drive" reconsidered. *J Hum Evol*. 1994; 26: 353–374.
40. Rollison J, Martin R. Comparative aspects of primate locomotion, with special reference to arboreal cercopithecines. *Symp Zool Soc Lond*. 1981; 48: 377–427.
41. Lovejoy C. The evolution of human walking. *Sci Am*. 1988; 259: 118–125.
42. Aiello L, Dean C. *An Introduction to Human Evolutionary Anatomy*. San Diego: Academic; 2002.
43. Fleagle J. *Primate Adaptations and Evolution*. San Diego: Academic; 1988/1999.
44. Whipple I. The ventral surface of the mammalian cheiridium, with special reference to the conditions found in man. *Z Morph Anthrop*. 1904; 7: 261–368.
45. Johnson R. Pads on the palm and sole of the human fetus. *Am Nat*. 1899; 33: 729–734.
46. Cartmill M. The volar skin of primates: Its frictional characteristics and their functional significance. *Am J Phys Anthropol*. 1979; 50: 497–510.
47. Hamrick M. Development and evolution of the mammalian limb: Adaptive diversification of nails, hooves, and claws. *Evol Devel*. 2001; 3: 355–363.
48. Szalay FS, Delson E. *Evolutionary History of the Primates*. New York: Academic; 1979.
49. Steiner H. Der Aufbau des Säugetier-Carpus und-Tarsus nach neueren embyologischen Untersuchungen. *Rev Suisse Zool*. 1942; 49: 217–223.
50. Cartmill M. Rethinking primate origins. *Science*. 1974; 184: 436–443.
51. Schmitt D, Lemelin P. Origins of primate locomotion: Gait mechanics of the woolly opossum. *Am J Phys Anthrop*. 2002; 118: 231–238.
52. Bloch J, Boyer D. Grasping primate origins. *Science*. 2002; 298: 1606–1610.
53. Conroy G. *Primate Evolution*. New York: W.W. Norton; 1990,
54. Szalay FS, Decker RL. Origins, evolution, and function of the tarsus in Late Cretaceous Eutheria and Paleocene primates. In: Jenkins FA, ed. *Primate Locomotion*, New York: Academic; 1974: 223–260.
55. Dagosto M. Postcranial anatomy and locomotor behavior in Eocene primates. In: Gebo D, ed. *Postcranial Adaptations in Nonhuman Primates*. DeKalb, IL: Northern Illinois University Press;1993:199–219.

56. Rasmussen D. Early catarrhines of the African Eocene and Oligocene. In: Hartwig W, ed. *The Primate Fossil Record*, Cambridge: Cambridge University Press; 2002.

57. Gebo D. Postcranial anatomy and locomotor adaptation in early African anthropoids. In: Gebo D, ed. *Postcranial Adaptations in Nonhuman Primates*, DeKalb, IL: Northern Illinois University Press; 1993b: 220–234.

58. Kay R, Fleagle J, Simons E. *A* revision of the Oligocene apes of Fayum Province, Egypt. *Am J Phys Anthrop*. 1981; 55: 293–322.

59. Fleagle J, Kay R. The phyletic position of *Parapithecidae. J Hum Evol*. 1987; 16: 483–532.

60. Andrews PJ. Family group systematics and evolution among catarrhine primates. In: Delson E, ed. *Ancestors: The Hard Evidence*. New York: Alan R. Liss; 1985: 14–22.

61. Harrison T. The phyletic relationships of the early catarrhine primates: A review of the current evidence. *J Hum Evol*. 1987; 16: 41–80.

62. Sarmiento E. The significance of the heel process in anthropoids. *Int J Primatol*. 1983; 4: 127–152.

63. Harrison T. *Late Oligocene to Middle Miocene Catarrhines from Afro-Arabia*. Hartwig W, ed. Cambridge: Cambridge University Press; 2002: 311–338.

64. Andrews PJ. Evolution and environment in the Hominoidea. *Nature*.1992; 360: 41–646.

65. Rose M. Locomotor anatomy of Miocene hominoids.In: Gebo D, ed. *Functional Morphology of the Foot in Primates*, 1993, DeKalb, IL: Northern Illinois University Press; 252–272.

66. Begun D, Teaford M, Walker A. Comparative and functional anatomy of *Proconsul* phalanges from the Kaswanga Primate Site, Rusinga Island, Kenya. *J Hum Evol*. 1994; 26: 89–165.

67. Langdon J. Functional morphology of the Miocene hominoid foot. In: *Contributions to Primatology*. Vol. 22. Szalay F, ed. New York: Karger; 1986,

68. Walker AC, Pickford M. New postcranial fossils of *Proconsul africanus* and *Proconsul nyanzae*. In: Ciochon RL, Corruccini RS, eds. *New Interpretations of Ape and Human Ancestry*. New York: Plenum;1983: 325–351.

69. Ishida H, et al. *Nacholapithecus* skeleton from the Middle Miocene of Kenya. *J. Hum. Evol*. 2004; 46: 69–103.

70. Begun D. European hominoids. In: Hartwig W, ed. *The Primate Fossil Record*. Cambridge: Cambridge University Press; 2002: 339–368.

71. Begun DR. New catarrhine phalanges from Rudabanya (Northeastern Hungary) and the problem of parallelism and convergence in the hominoid postcranial morphology. *J Human Evol*. 1993a; 24: 373–402.

72. Tuttle R. Knuckle-walking and the problem of human origins. *Science*. 1969;166: 953–961.

73. Tuttle R. Darwin's apes, dental apes, and the descent of man: normal science in evolutionary anthropology. *Curr Anthrop*.1974;15: 389–398.

74. Stern J. Before bipedality. *Yrbk Phys Anthrop*. 1975; 19: 59–68.

75. Prost, J., Origin of bipedalism. *Am J Phys Anthrop*. 1980; 52: 175–189.

76. Fleagle J, et al. Climbing: A biomechanical link with brachiation and bipedalism. *Symp Zool Soc Lond*. 1981; 48: 359–373.

77. Stern J, Susman R. Electromyography of the gluteal muscles in *Hylobates*, *Pongo*, and *Pan*: Implications for the evolution of hominid bipedality. *Am J Phys Anthrop*. 1981; 55: 153–166.

78. Ishida H, Kumakura H, Kondo S.Primate bipedalism and quadrupedalism: comparative electromyography. In: Kondo S, ed. *Primate Morphophysiology, Locomotor Analyses and Human Bipedalism*, Tokyo: University of Tokyo Press; 1985: 59–79.

79. Senut B. Climbing as a crucial preadaptation for human bipedalism. *Int J Skeletal Res*. 1988; 14: 35–44.

80. Gebo D. Climbing, brachiation, and terrestrial quadrupedalism: historical precursors of hominid bipedalism. *Am J Phys Anthrop*. 1996; 101: 55–92.

81. Sarmiento E. Generalized quadrupeds, committed bipeds and the shift to open habitats: An evolutionary model of hominid divergence. *Am Mus Novitates*. 1998; 3250: 1–78.
82. Washburn S. Behavior and the origin of Man. *Proc R Anthrop Inst Gr Br Ire*. 1967; 3: 21–27.
83. Corruccini R. Comparative osteometrics of the hominoid wrist joint, with special reference to knuckle-walking. *J Human Evol*.1978; 7: 307–321.
84. Shea B, Inouye S. Knuckle-walking ancestors. *Science*. 1993; 259: 293–294.
85. Begun D. Knuckle-walking ancestors. *Science*. 1993b. 259: 294.
86. Begun D. Relations among the great apes and humans: new interpretations based on the fossil great ape *Dryopithecus*. *Yrbk Phys Anthrop*. 1994; 37: 11–63.
87. Richmond B, Strait D. Evidence that humans evolved from a knuckle-walking ancestor. *Nature*. 2000; 404: 382–385.
88. Richmond B, Begun D, Strait D. Origin of human bipedalism: The knuckle-walking hypothesis revisited. *Am J Phys Anthrop*. 2001; 44: 70–105.
89. Gebo D. Plantigrady and foot adaptation in African apes: implications for hominid evolution. *Am J Phys Anthrop*. 1992; 89: 29–58.
90. Meldrum D. On plantigrady and quadrupedalism. *Am J Phys Anthrop*. 1993; 91: 379–381.
91. Schmitt D, Larson S. Heel contact as a function of substrate type and speed in primates. *Am J Phys Anthrop*. 1995; 96: 39–50.
92. Horai S, et al. Recent African origin of modern humans revealed by complete sequences of hominoid mitochondrial DNAs. *Proc Nat Acad Sci USA*.1995; 92: 532–536.
93. Ruvolo M. Molecular phylogeny of the hominoids: Inferences from multiple independent DNA sequence data sets. *Mol Biol Evol*. 1997; 14: 248–265.
94. Chen F-C, Li W-H. Genomic divergences between humans and other hominoids and the effective population size of the common ancestor of humans and chimpanzees. *Am J Hum Genetics*. 2001; 68: 444–456.
95. Brunet M, et al. A new hominid from the upper Miocene of Chad, Central Africa. *Nature*. 2002; 418: 145–151.
96. Wolpoff M, et al. *Sahelanthropus* or *'Sahelpithecus'? Nature*. 2002; 419: 581–582.
97. Senut B, et al. First hominid from the Miocene (Lukeino Formation, Kenya). *CR Acad Sci*. 2001; 332: 137–144.
98. Ward S, Duren D. Middle and late Miocene African hominoids. In Hartwig W, ed. *The Primate Fossil Record*, Cambridge: Cambridge University Press; 2002: 385–397.
99. Haile-Selassie Y. Late Miocene hominids from the Middle Awash, Ethiopia. *Nature*. 2001; 412: 178–181.
100. Galick K, et al. External and internal morphology of the BAR 1002′ 00 *Orrorin tugenensis* femur. *Science*. 2004; 1450–1453.
101. Coates, M.I. and Clack, J.A. 1995. Romer's Gap – Tetrapod origins and terrestriality. In: Arsenault M, Lelivre H, Janvier P, eds. Proceedings of the 7th International Symposium on Early Vertebrates. *Bulletin du Muséum national d'Histoire naturelle, Paris*. 373–388.
102. Adams LA, Eddy, S. 1949. *Comparative Anatomy*. 2d ed. London: Chapman & Hall.
103. Lewis O.J. The homologies of the mammalian tarsal bones. *J Anat*. 1964; 98.
104. Kirk EC, et al. Comment on "Grasping Primate Origins". *Science*. 2003; 300:741.

2
Recent Evolution of the Human Foot

This chapter deals with the recent evolution of the human foot. Its scope is more limited than Chapter 1. Instead of spanning approximately 400 million years it covers only 8 million years, and instead of dealing with the vertebrate branch of the Tree of Life it considers just one of the many small terminal twigs, or clades, that make up the primate part of the Tree of Life. We focus on a series of extinct mammals called hominins that through time, and in fits and starts, accumulate morphology more similar to modern humans and less like that of the other great apes. Researchers have differing views about how many branches the twig has, and they also disagree about how reliably we are able to reconstruct the branching pattern within the twig. We try to reflect these different views in our discussion.

This chapter has three sections. The first provides an overview of the hominin fossil record. We use a relatively complex taxonomic hypothesis consistent with human evolution being interpreted as a series of closely related branches called adaptive radiations. A second simpler taxonomic hypothesis that interprets human evolution as a more 'ladderlike' progression is presented in summary form.

The second section of the chapter reviews hypotheses about the evolution of hominin bipedal locomotion. This focuses on scenarios put forward to explain the origin of bipedalism, and on debates about whether bipedalism evolved once, or several times, within the hominin clade.

The third section reviews each hominin taxon, focusing on what is known about the foot. Most of this information is gleaned from fossil foot bones that have, with varying degrees of certainty, been assigned to hominin taxa. However, other information has come from so-called 'trace fossils,' which are the impressions made by the feet of early hominins.

Hominin Evolution: An Overview

Terminology

For reasons given below we treat modern humans as one of the 'great apes', the other three being the two African great apes, chimpanzee (*Pan*) and the gorilla (*Gorilla*), and the only Asian great ape, the orangutan (*Pongo*).

Palaeoanthropologists have differed, and still do differ in the way they classify the higher primates. We have tried to avoid technical terms in this section, but some are necessary in order to understand the implications of the different classifications.

Chapter co-written by Nicole L. Griffin.

Linnaean taxonomic categories immediately above the level of the genus, that is, the family and the tribe, have vernacular equivalents that end in 'id' and 'in', respectively. In the past *Homo sapiens* has been considered to be distinct enough to be placed in its own family, the Hominidae, with the other great apes grouped together in a separate family, the Pongidae. Thus, modern humans and their close fossil relatives were referred to as 'hominids', and the other great apes and their close fossil relatives were referred to as 'pongids' (Table 2.1A). However, this scheme is inconsistent with morphological and genetic evidence suggesting modern humans are more closely related to chimpanzees than they are to either gorillas or orangutans.

In response to the overwhelming evidence that modern humans and chimpanzees are more closely related to each other than either is to the gorilla or the orangutan, some researchers advocate combining modern humans and chimps in the same genus (e.g., [1]), which according to the rules of zoological nomenclature must be *Homo*. We adopt a less radical solution. We lump all the great apes into a single family, the Hominidae (Table 2.1B). Within the Hominidae we recognise three subfamilies, the Ponginae for the orangutans, the Gorillinae for the gorillas, and the Homininae for modern humans and chimpanzees. The latter subfamily is broken down into two tribes, Panini (or 'panins') for chimpanzees, and Hominini (or 'hominins') for modern humans. The latter is further broken down into two subtribes: one, Australopithecina, for the extinct primitive hominin genera, and the other, Hominina for the genus *Homo*, which includes the only living hominin taxon, *Homo sapiens*. Modern humans and all the fossil taxa judged to be more closely related to modern humans than to chimpanzees are called 'hominins'; the chimpanzee equivalent is 'panin'. Thus, modern humans are 'hominids' (family), 'hominines' (subfamily), and then 'hominins' (tribe). We use 'australopith' when we refer to taxa belonging to the subtribe Australopithecina.

Defining Hominins

Molecular biology has revolutionised our knowledge of the relationships within the great ape clade of the Tree of Life. Relationships between organisms can now be pursued at the level of the genome instead of having to rely on morphology (traditional hard and/or soft-tissue anatomy or the morphology of proteins) for information about relatedness. Comparisons of the DNA of organisms have been made using two methods. In DNA hybridisation all the DNA is compared, but at a relatively crude level. In DNA sequencing the base sequences of comparable sections of DNA are determined and then compared. The results of both hybridisation (e.g., [2]) and sequencing studies of both nuclear and mtDNA (e.g., [1,3,4–6]) are virtually unanimous in suggesting that modern humans and the two African apes are more closely related to each other than any of them is to the orangutan. They also suggest that modern humans and modern chimpanzees (belonging to the genus *Pan*) are more closely related to each other than either is to the gorilla.

Table 1   'Old' and 'New' Taxonomies

(A) A traditional 'premolecular' taxonomy of higher primates. Extinct taxa are in bold.
Superfamily Hominoidea (hominoids)
   Family Hylobatidae (hylobatids)
      Genus *Hylobates*
   Family Pongidae (pongids)
      Genus *Pongo*
      Genus *Gorilla*
      Genus *Pan*
   Family Hominidae (hominids)
      Subfamily **Australopithecinae (australopithecines)**
         Genus ***Ardipithecus***
         Genus ***Australopithecus***
         Genus ***Kenyanthropus***
         Genus ***Orrorin***
         Genus ***Paranthropus***
         Genus ***Sahelanthropus***
     Subfamily Homininae (hominines)
        Genus *Homo*

(B) A taxonomy of higher primates that recognizes the close genetic links between *Pan* and
   Homo. Extinct taxa are in bold type.
Superfamily Hominoidea (hominoids)
   Family Hylobatidae (hylobatids)
      Genus *Hylobates*
   Family Hominidae (hominids)
      Subfamily Ponginae
         Genus *Pongo* (pongines)
      Subfamily Gorillinae
         Genus *Gorilla* (gorillines)
      Subfamily Homininae (hominines)
        Tribe Panini
          Genus *Pan* (panins)
        Tribe Hominini (hominins)
         Subtribe Australopithecina (australopiths)
           Genus ***Ardipithecus***
           Genus ***Australopithecus***
           Genus ***Kenyanthropus***
           Genus ***Orrorin***
           Genus ***Paranthropus***
           Genus ***Sahelanthropus***
         Subtribe Hominina (hominans)
          Genus *Homo*

Most attempts to predict the date of the *Pan/Homo* dichotomy suggest that the hypothetical ancestor of modern humans and chimpanzees lived between about 5 and 8 Mya (e.g., [7]), but some researchers (e.g., [8]) favour a substantially earlier date (10–14 Mya) for the divergence of the *Pan* and *Homo* lineages.

Thus, if we accept that the hominin twig of the Tree of Life may extend back in time to ca. 8 Mya, and that the earliest unambiguous hominin is probably *Australopithecus anamensis* (see below), then between 8 and 4 Mya we would expect to find primitive hominin and primitive panin taxa, and close to 8 Mya we should expect to see evidence of the common ancestor of panins and hominins. Not all of these taxa are direct ancestors of modern humans and chimpanzees; many will belong to extinct panin and hominin subclades. Some of these taxa could also belong to extinct clades that have yet to be recognised in the fossil record.

Organising the Hominin Fossil Record

The classification of the hominin fossil evidence is controversial. Some researchers favour recognising relatively few taxa, whereas others think that more species and genera are needed to accommodate the observed morphological diversity. We use a relatively speciose (or 'splitting') taxonomy, but we also provide an example of a less speciose (or 'lumping') taxonomy so that readers can appreciate how the evidence for human evolution would look if it were interpreted in a different way. The taxa included in the two taxonomies are listed in Table 2.2. Some of the taxon names are used in different senses in the speciose and less-speciose taxonomies. When we refer in the text to the hypodigm (the fossil evidence referred to that taxon) of one of these taxa in the speciose taxonomy we use the taxon name followed by *sensu stricto* (e.g., *Au. afarensis sensu stricto* or its abbreviation, *Au. afarensis s. s.*). This signifies that we are using the taxon name in its 'strict' sense. When we refer to the same taxon in the more inclusive taxonomy (i.e., the hypodigm is larger) the Linnaean binomial is followed by *sensu lato* (e.g., *Au. afarensis sensu lato* or *Au. afarensis s. l.*). This indicates we are using the taxon name in a 'looser' sense. To save repetition, and because in most cases we are referring to the taxa in their strict sense, readers should assume we mean *sensu stricto* unless we specifically refer to *sensu lato*, or use *s. l.*

The temporal spans of the taxa in the speciose taxonomy are illustrated in Table 2.2 and Figure 2.1. The ages of the first and last appearances of any taxon in the fossil record (called the 'first appearance datum' or FAD, and 'last appearance datum' or LAD, respectively) almost certainly underestimate the temporal range of the taxa. Nonetheless, FADs and LADs provide an approximate temporal sequence for the hominin taxa. The heights of the columns of those taxa with good, well-dated, fossil records (e.g., *Australopithecus afarensis* and *Paranthropus boisei*) are a reasonable estimate of the temporal range of those taxa, but the heights of the columns for the taxa marked with an asterisk (e.g., *Sahelanthropus tchadensis* and *Australopithecus bahrelghazali*) reflect uncertainties about the age

Table 2 Splitting and lumping hominin taxonomies and skeletal representation[1] of splitting hominin taxa

Informal group	A. Splitting taxonomy	Age (Ma)	Type specimen	Crania	Dentition	Axial	Upper limb	Lower limb
Primitive hominins	S. tchadensis*	7.0 – 6.0	TM 266-01-060-1	X	X			X
	O. tugenensis*	6.0	BAR 1000'00	X	X		X	ff
	Ar. ramidus s.s*	5.7 – 4.5	ARA-VP-6/1	X	X		X	X
	Ar. kadabba*	5.8 – 5.2	ALA-VP-2/10		X		X	X
Archaic hominins	Au. anamensis*	4.5 – 4.0	KNM-KP 29281	ff	X		X	X
	Au. afarensis s. s.	4.0 – 3.0	LH 4	X	X	X	X	
	K. platyops*	3.5 – 3.3	KNM-WT 40000	X	X			
	Au. bahrelghazali*	3.5 – 3.0	KT 12/H1		X			
	Au. africanus*	3.0 – 2.4	Taung 1	X	X	X	X	X
Megadont archaic hominins	Au. garhi*	2.5	BOU-VP-12/130	X	X		?	?
	P. aethiopicus*	2.5 – 2.3	Omo 18.18	X	X			
	P. boisei s. s.	2.3 – 1.3	OH 5	X	X		?	?
	P. robustus*	2.0 – 1.5	TM 1517	X	X		X	X
Archaic Homo	H. habilis s. s.*	2.4 – 1.6	OH 7	X	X	X	X	X
	H. rudolfensis*	2.4 – 1.6	KNM-ER 1470	X	X			?
	H. ergaster*	1.9 – 1.5	KNM-ER 992	X	X	X	X	X
	H. erectus s. s.	1.8 – 0.2	Trinil 2	X	X		X	X
	H. floresiensis [3]	0.095 – 0.018	LB1	X	X	ff	ff	X
	H. antecessor*	0.7 – 0.5	ATD6-5	X	X			
	H. heidelbergensis	0.6 – 0.1	Mauer 1	X	X		ff	X
	H. neander thalensis	0.2 – 0.03	Neanderthal 1	X	X	X	X	X
Anatomically-modern Homo	H. sapiens s. s.	0.16 -pres	None designated	X	X	X	X	X

(Continued)

Table 2 *(Continued)*

Informal group	**B.** Lumping taxonomy	Age (Ma)	Taxa included from splitting taxonomy
Primitive hominins	*Ar. ramidus s. l.**	7.0 – 4.5	*Ar. ramidus s. s., Ar. kadabba, S. tchadensis, O. tugenensis*
Archaic hominins	*Au. afarensis s. l.*	4.5 – 3.0	*Au. afarensis s. s., Au. anamensis, Au. bahrelghazali, K. platyops*
	*Au. africanus**	3.0 – 2.4	*Au. africanus*
Megadont archaic hominins	*P. boisei s. l.*	2.5 – 1.3	*P. boisei s. s., P. aethiopicus, Au. garhi*
	*P. robustus**	2.0 – 1.5	*P. robustus*
Archaic *Homo*	*H. habilis s. l.**	2.4 – 1.6	*H. habilis s. s., H. rudolfensis*
	H. erectus s. l.	1.9 – 0.018	*H. erectus s. s., H. ergaster, H. floresiensis*
Anatomically-modern *Homo*	*H. sapiens s. l.*	0.7 -pres	*H. sapiens s. s., H. antecessor, H. heidelbergensis, H. neanderthalensis*

Notes:
1. Skeletal representation key: X – present; ff -fragmentary specimens; ? -taxonomic affiliation of fossil specimen(s) uncertain.

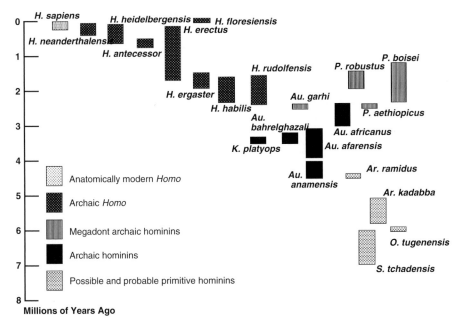

Figure 2.1. Speciose hominin taxonomy.

of the taxon because either the sample size is too small, or because the dating methods used are imprecise.

For various reasons it is very unlikely that we have a complete record of hominin taxonomic diversity, particularly in the pre-4 Mya phase of hominin evolution. This is because intensive explorations of sediments of this age have only been conducted for less than a decade, and because these investigations have been restricted in their geographical scope. Thus, the fossil evidence we are working with in the early phase of hominin evolution is almost certainly incomplete. More taxa are likely to be identified. We should bear this in mind when formulating and testing hypotheses about any aspect of hominin evolution, especially the evolution of bipedalism. We have not used lines to connect the taxa in the most likely ancestor-descendent sequence, we are reluctant to do this because the constraints of existing knowledge suggest there are only two relatively well-supported subclades within the hominin clade, one for *Paranthropus* taxa and the other for post-*Homo ergaster* taxa belonging to the *Homo* clade. Without more well-supported subclades it is probably unwise to begin to try to identify specific taxa as ancestors or descendants of other taxa. The taxa in Table 2.2 have been assigned to five relatively crude grades [9]; these are based on brain size, postcanine tooth size, and inferred locomotor mode. Several taxon samples are too small to do other than make an informed guess about the grade of the taxon.

Evolution of Bipedalism within the Hominin Clade

One of the most important discoveries relevant to palaeoanthropology in the past century or so has nothing to do with the fossil record. It is the recognition that the chimpanzee genome is more similar to the modern human genome than it is to the genome of the gorilla [10]. This means that the ancestor of all later hominins is itself a descendant of the common ancestor of chimpanzees and hominins. Thus, if we could make reliable inferences about the posture and locomotion of the chimp/human common ancestor this would help narrow down the options for the posture and locomotion of the earliest members of the hominin clade.

As we have seen in Chapter 1, comparative evidence suggests that the foot of the chimp/human common ancestor was already adapted for plantigrade loco-motion. This is a form of locomotion in which the heel is the first part of the foot to strike the ground at the end of the swing phase [11]. The principle of parsimony suggests that the foot of the chimp/human common ancestor would be more similar to that of living chimpanzees than to the modern human foot. Thus, when seen in the context of the other higher primates it is the posture and loco-motion of modern humans that is unusual, not that of chimpanzees. Chimpanzees mostly climb and walk quadrupedally on large branches when they are in the trees. They do brachiate, but it is a minor part of their arboreal behaviour. For most of the time they are on the ground they are quadrupedal knuckle-walkers; bipedal terrestrial locomotion is rare (Figure 2.2). The tarsal bones of modern chimpanzees reflect this locomotor mix. The talus has a moderately long neck, an asymmetrical trochlear surface, the calcaneocuboid joint is designed for rotation, and the transverse tarsal joints are designed for mobility. More distally the hallux is abducted and opposable, and the long and curved phalanges have prominent flexor sheath ridges. We predict these traits will be among those possessed by the foot of the chimp/human common ancestor.

Rose [12] points out that among primates, and especially higher primates, modern humans are unusual because they are committed to a single locomotor mode. Whereas other primates have a locomotor repertoire made up of several locomotor strategies, modern humans have only one locomotor strategy or mode. This is the form of locomotion we call *obligate bipedalism*. For example, in modern chimpanzees the two major locomotor strategies employed are climbing and quadrupedal knuckle-walking, with brachiation and bipedalism playing progressively smaller roles in the locomotor repertoire of chimpanzees. Higher primates that have the ability, or facility, to move bipedally are called *facultative bipeds*, and Rose [12] predicts that in the common ancestor of chimps/humans facultative bipedalism would have established itself as the third major component of its locomotor repertoire, along with climbing and knuckle-walking (Figure 2.3). What we presently do not know is whether this hypothesised relatively modest increase in emphasis on bipedalism was confined to the hominin clade, or whether it also

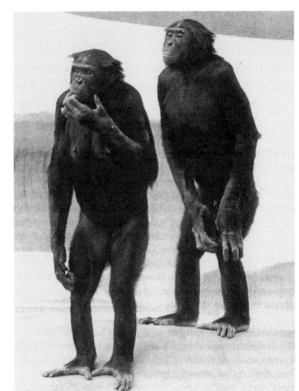

Figure 2.2. Bipedal postures of bonobos (pygmy chimpanzees). These close relatives of humans are only infrequent bipeds; they mainly locomote quadrupedally or by climbing. Note the absence of a longitudinal arch, the divergent or abducted hallux, and the long toes. It is predicted that the chimp/human common ancestor and the earliest hominins would have had similar feet. (From Bernard G. Campbell, James D. Loy. Humankind Emerging, 7/e. Published by Allyn and Bacon, Boston, MA. Copyright © 1996 by Pearson Education. Reprinted by permission of the publisher.)

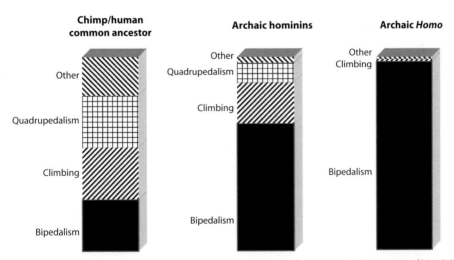

Figure 2.3. Proposed early hominin locomotor repertoires. (Adapted from Rose MD. *The process of bipedalization in hominds*, in *Origine(s) de la Bipédie Chez les Hominidés*, Y. Coppens and B. Senut, Editors. 1991, Centre National de la Recherche Scientifique: Paris. p. 40.)

occurred in any nonhominin clade. We also do not know whether this increased emphasis on bipedalism occurred just once within the hominin clade, or whether it occurred independently in an extinct higher primate clade, or in more than one hominin subclade. For various reasons, most researchers consider it is likely that any increase in the importance of facultative bipedalism in early hominins would have been at the cost of quadrupedal locomotion.

Scenarios Favouring Selection for Bipedalism

Scenarios explaining the origin of bipedalism can be divided into those that necessitate the adoption of bipedalism as the predominant locomotor mode, and those that favour the adoption of bipedalism. Scenarios that necessitate bipedalism include all the models that involve: (1) the forelimbs being used for prolonged periods for purposes other than locomotion, or (2) the forelimbs being used for any period, short or long, which requires sufficiently radical changes in morphology that they reduce the efficiency of the hands for quadrupedal loco-motion or for climbing. The scenarios that necessitate bipedal locomotion include the carriage of infants, food, or tools. The scenarios that favour bipedal locomotion include fast running to evade predators, and more efficient long dis-tance travel between resources that are widely distributed in patches (Figure 2.4).

It is also possible that an increased emphasis on an upright, or bipedal, posture may have been an important stimulus for the adoption of a locomotor strategy that included a higher proportion of bipedal locomotion. For example, scenarios that would have favoured an upright bipedal posture include: (1) a shift to a habi-

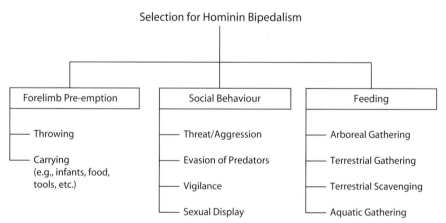

Figure 2.4. The three categories, forelimb pre-emption, social behaviour, and feeding may have influenced the adoption of bipedalism by hominins. (Adapted from Rose MD. *The process of bipedalization in hominds*, in *Origine(s) de la Bipédie Chez les Hominidés*, Y. Coppens and B. Senut, Editors. 1991, Centre National de la Recherche Scientifique: Paris. p. 41.)

tat in which being upright has advantages for thermoregulation [13]; (2) the use of an upright posture for displays, threats, and aggression [14,15]; or (3) the use of an upright posture for arboreal feeding [16]. It is, of course, possible and likely that at any one time more than one of these influences was operating to increase the Darwinian fitness of the members of early hominin taxa that opted to increase the proportion of bipedal travel in their locomotor repertoire. It is also likely that more than one of the influences reviewed above may have been involved at different times during the evolution of early hominin facultative bipedalism.

Of all the scenarios that have been put forward for its evolution, the hypothesis that obligate bipedalism is a byproduct of selection for manual dexterity is the most appealing. But as can be seen from the review above, once an upright posture and a bipedal gait had been incorporated into the locomotor repertoire of a hominin taxon, then other factors may well have contributed to it assuming an increasing importance in that locomotor repertoire until eventually facultative bipedalism progressed to obligate bipedalism.

Almost all discussions of hominin bipedal locomotion usually make the implicit assumption that early hominins were adapted for bipedal walking. However, two researchers have recently revived an earlier proposal [17] that the selection may have been not for walking, but for bipedal endurance running [18]. The authors suggest that several of the morphological features of the modern human foot are more easily explained as adaptations to running than to walking (*ibid.*, 347). At present the earliest evidence of obligate bipedalism within the hominin clade is seen in *Homo ergaster*, or East African *Homo erectus*. Most researchers take the view that hominin obligate bipedalism involves such a complicated set of adjustments to the postcranial skeleton that it is unlikely to have occurred more than once. However, there is good evidence that many hominin adaptations may be homoplasies; that is, they were not inherited from a recent common ancestor. There is also no reason to think that the morphology associated with posture and locomotion is any less prone to homoplasy than, say, the morphology associated with mastication. Thus, it would be unwise to categorically exclude the possibility that facultative bipedalism, or even obligate bipedalism could have evolved more than once in the hominin clade. Therefore we should be cautious before assuming that all later bipedal hominin taxa, be they facultative or obligate bipeds, necessarily inherited their bipedal adaptations from a common ancestor.

Review of Individual Hominin Fossil Taxa

Each hominin taxon is placed in one of five informal groupings, 'primitive hominins' (P), 'archaic hominins' (A), 'megadont archaic hominins' (M), 'archaic *Homo*' (AH), and 'anatomically-modern *Homo*' (H) (Table 2.2). Within each grouping the taxa are listed in order of their first appearance in the fossil record.

Unless homoplasy (shared morphology not derived from the most recent common ancestor) is even more common than we anticipate, there is little doubt that recent hominin taxa [i.e., post-*H. ergaster* taxa in group (AH)] are more closely related to modern humans than to chimpanzees. These taxa all have absolutely and relatively large brains; they were obligate bipeds; and they have small canines, slender jaws, and small chewing teeth. However, the closer we get to the split between hominins and panins the more difficult it is to find features we can be sure fossil hominins possessed and fossil panins, or taxa in any other closely-related clade, did not. In the early stages of hominin evolution it may be either the lack of panin features or relatively subtle differences in the size and shape of the canines, or in the detailed morphology of the limbs, that mark out hominins.

We are conscious that many readers of this book may be unfamiliar with the details of the hominin fossil record, so we provide basic information about the morphology of each taxon. We have deliberately not sorted these features into 'primitive' (or plesiomorphic), 'derived' (or synapomorphic), and 'unique' (or autapomorphic) because this would suggest that hominin cladograms are more reliable than we believe them to be. When a taxon has been moved from its initial genus, the original reference is given in parentheses followed by the revising reference. Further details about most of the taxa and a more extensive bibliography can be found in Wood and Richmond [19]; only selected recent references are cited here. Recent relevant reviews of most of these taxa can be found in Hartwig [20] and Wood and Constantino [21].

Modern and prehistoric carnivores are, and apparently were, partial to hands and feet. Thus there are relatively few hand and foot bones in the hominin fossil record. Clearly this changes when corpses were deliberately buried, but this did not occur until relatively recently, probably within the last 100 Kya.

Some hominin fossil foot bones have been found at sites where there is cranial evidence for more than one hominin taxon (e.g., the 2.2 Mya calcaneum, Omo 33.74.896 and the 2.36 Mya talus, Omo 323-76-898, both from the Omo Shungura Formation, two tali, KNM-ER 1464 and 1476, from Koobi Fora and the 1.8 Mya foot fossils from Swartkrans). Because it is impossible to be sure which of the hominin taxa known from these sites these fossil foot bones belong to, we have not included evidence about these remains in any of the taxa listed below.

A note about the dates provided for the taxa. Age estimates are given in either millions (Mya) or thousands (Kya) of years.

Primitive Hominins

This category includes one taxon, *Ardipithecus ramidus*, that is almost certainly a member of the hominin clade, one taxon, *Sahelanthropus tchadensis*, that is a probable hominin, and two taxa, *Ardipithecus kadabba* and *Orrorin tugenensis*, that may be hominins.

Taxon name: Sahelanthropus tchadensis Brunet et al., 2001.

Temporal range: ca. 7–6 Mya.

Source(s) of the evidence: Toros-Menalla, Chad, Central Africa.

Nature of the evidence: A distorted cranium, several mandibles, and some teeth; no postcranial evidence.

Characteristics and inferred behaviour: A chimp-sized animal displaying a novel combination of primitive and derived features. Much about the base and vault of the cranium is chimplike, but the relatively anterior placement of the foramen magnum, the presence of a supraorbital torus, the lack of a muzzle, the small, apically-worn canines, the low, rounded, molar cusps, the relatively thick tooth enamel, and the relatively thick mandibular corpus [22] suggest that *S. tchadensis* does not belong in the *Pan* clade. It is either a primitive hominin, or it belongs to a separate, but closely-related, clade of homininlike apes.

Pedal fossil evidence: None.

Taxon name: Orrorin tugenensis Senut et al., 2001.

Temporal range: ca. 6 Mya.

Source(s) of the evidence: The relevant remains come from four localities in the Lukeino Formation, Tugen Hills, Kenya.

Nature of the evidence: The 13 specimens include three femoral fragments.

Characteristics and inferred behaviour: The femoral morphology has been interpreted [24,25] as suggesting that *O. tugenensis* is an obligate biped, but other researchers interpret the radiographs and CT scans of the femoral neck as indicating a mix of bipedal and nonbipedal locomotion. Otherwise, the discoverers admit that much of the critical dental morphology is 'ape-like' [26, p. 6]. *O. tugenensis* may prove to be a hominin, but it is more likely that it belongs to another part of the adaptive radiation that included the common ancestor of panins and hominins.

Pedal fossil evidence: None.

Taxon name: Ardipithecus kadabba, Haile-Selassie et al., 2004.

Temporal range: 5.8–5.2 Mya.

Source(s) of the evidence: Middle Awash, Ethiopia.

Nature of the evidence: Mandible, teeth, and postcranial evidence.

Characteristics and inferred behaviour: The upper canine and lower first premolar morphology is less apelike than that of *O. tugenensis*, but more apelike than that of *Ar. ramidus*. The researchers who found it suggest that it 'closely approaches the extant and fossil ape condition' [26, p. 1505], and they also suggest that the morphology of the canine–premolar complex of *S. tchadensis*, *O. tugenensis*, and *Ar. kadabba* is so similar that they may belong to one genus, or even one species (*ibid.*).

Pedal fossil evidence: The only evidence of the foot is a 5.2 Mya fourth proximal phalanx. Haile-Selassie [27] suggests the curvature, length, and dorsal-canting of the proximal articular surface are traits shared with the Pliocene hominin, *Au. afarensis*. Richmond et al. [28] caution against treating the latter trait as evidence of bipedalism because Duncan et al. [29] did not find a significant difference between the proximal articular surface shape of *Au. afarensis* and quadrupedal primates such as the African apes.

Taxon name: Ardipithecus ramidus sensu stricto (White et al., 1994) White et al. 1995.

Temporal range: ca. 4.5–4.4 Mya.

Source(s) of the evidence: The initial evidence for this taxon came from a site called Aramis in the Middle Awash region of Ethiopia. A second suite of fossils, including a mandible, teeth, and postcranial bones, recovered in 1997 from five different localities in the Middle Awash that range in age from 5.2–<5.7 Mya were initially allocated to this taxon [27], but they were subsequently transferred to *Ar. kadabba* (see above). Hominins dating from between 4.5 and 4.3 Mya from a site called As Duma, in Gona, near Hadar, Ethiopia, have recently been added to the hypodigm [32].

Nature of the evidence: The published evidence consists of isolated teeth, a piece of the base of the cranium, and fragments of mandibles and long bones. A fragmented associated skeleton has been found and is being prepared and reconstructed.

Characteristics and inferred behaviour: The remains attributed to *Ar. ramidus* share some features in common with living species of *Pan*, others that are shared with the African apes in general, and, crucially, several dental and cranial features that are shared only with later hominins such as *Au. afarensis*. The discoverers initially allocated the new species to *Australopithecus* [30], but they subsequently assigned it to a new genus, *Ardipithecus* [31]. Judging from the size of the shoulder joint *Ar. ramidus* weighed about 40 kg. Its chewing teeth were relatively small and the position of the foramen magnum suggests that the posture and gait of *Ar. ramidus* were, respectively, more upright and bipedal than is the case in the living apes. The thin enamel covering on the teeth suggests that the diet of *Ar. ramidus* may have been closer to that of the chimpanzee than to modern humans.

Pedal fossil evidence: The proximal third of a pedal phalanx (GWM1/P37) has been recovered from the As Duma site and is between 4.5 and 4.3 million years old. GWM1/P37 has a dorsally canted proximal articular facet that is similar to those belonging to *Ar. kadabba* and *Au. afarensis* [32].

Archaic Hominins

This group includes all the hominin taxa assigned to the two genera, *Australopithecus* and *Kenyanthropus*. As it is used in this and many other taxonomies *Australopithecus* is almost certainly not a single clade, but until researchers can generate a reliable phylogeny there is little point in revising its generic terminology.

Taxon name: Australopithecus anamensis Leakey et al. 1995.

Approximate time range: ca. 4.0–4.5 Mya.

Source(s) of the evidence: Allia Bay and Kanapoi, Kenya.

Nature of the evidence: The evidence consists of jaws, teeth, and postcranial elements from the upper and lower limbs.

Characteristics and inferred behaviour: The main differences between *Au. anamensis* and *Au. afarensis* relate to details of the dentition. In some respects the teeth of *Au. anamensis* are more primitive than those of *Au. afarensis* (e.g., the asymmetry of the premolar crowns and the relatively simple crowns of the deciduous first mandibular molars), but in others (e.g., the low cross-sectional profiles and bulging sides of the molar crowns) they show similarities to *Paranthropus* (see below). The upper limb remains are australopith-like, but a tibia attributed to *Au. anamensis* has features associated with bipedality.
Pedal fossil evidence: None.

Taxon name: Australopithecus afarensis sensu stricto Johanson et al. 1978.

Approximate time range: ca. 4–3 Mya.

Source(s) of the evidence: Laetoli, Tanzania; White Sands, Hadar, Maka, Belohdelie and Fejej, Ethiopia; Allia Bay, West Turkana and Tabarin, Kenya.

Nature of the evidence: Au. afarensis is the earliest hominin to have a comprehensive fossil record including a skull, fragmented skulls, many lower jaws, and sufficient limb bones to be able to estimate stature and body mass. The collection includes a specimen, AL-288, that preserves just less than half of the skeleton of an adult female.

Characteristics and inferred behaviour: The range of body mass estimates is from 25 to <50 kg. and the estimated endocranial volume of *Au. afarensis* is between 400 to 500 cm^3. This is larger than the average endocranial volume of a chimpanzee, but if the estimates of the body size of *Au. afarensis* are approximately correct, then relative to estimated body mass the brain of *Au. afarensis* is not substantially larger than that of *Pan*. It has incisors that are much smaller than those of extant chimpanzees, but the premolars and molars of *Au. afarensis* are relatively larger than those of the chimpanzee. The hind limbs of AL-288 are substantially shorter than those of a modern human of similar stature. The upper limb, especially the hand, retains morphology that most likely reflects a significant element of arboreal locomotion. The size of the footprints, the length of the stride, and stature estimates based on the length of the limb bones suggest that the standing height of adult individuals in this early hominin species was between 1.0 and 1.5 m.

Pedal fossil evidence:

Talus: Lewis [35] considers the form of the trochlear surface, especially the elevation of the anterior region of its lateral border, the laterally-flared lateral malleolus, and the anterior cuplike depression of the medial malleolus to be apelike features. In contrast, Latimer et al. [36] claim that the vertical orientation of the medial and lateral posterior talar tubercles, and the direction of the 'talocrural rotational axis' (the line connecting the two points of minimal motion of the medial and lateral surfaces of the talus) which in *Au. afarensis* is perpendicular to the long axis of the joint (Figure 2.5) are both evidence that plantarflexion was more restricted in *Au. afarensis* than in the African apes. Other features of the *Au. afarensis* talus that suggest decreased mobility of the ankle joint are its flatter trochlear surface and straighter medial border [11,36]. However, several researchers suggest that the range of plantar and dorsiflexion at the *Au. afarensis* ankle joint would have exceeded that of modern humans [36–39]. Gomberg and Latimer [40] describe the talonavicular joint of *Au. afarensis* as more mobile than in humans. Although Lamy [41] suggested the AL 288-1 talar head does not display the same degree of dorsolateral tilting as found in modern humans, Langdon et al. [42] found that the tilt of the head was within the range found in modern humans.

Calcaneum: There is disagreement about whether the morphology of the *Au. afarensis* calcaneum provides information about the existence of a longitudinal arch. In the human foot, this arch is associated with a strong calcaneal plantar tubercle [38,43]. Some researchers suggest that *Au. afarensis* shows evidence of a plantar tubercle [11,44,45], but others claim the tubercle is not well-enough developed to provide unambiguous evidence of a longitudinal arch [37,38], and Deloison [47] regards it as absent. Most researchers agree that the *Au. afarensis* calcaneum does have a substantial fibular trochlea [37,38,44,47,48], although Latimer

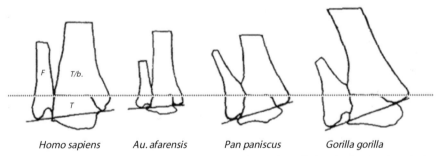

Homo sapiens   Au. afarensis   Pan paniscus   Gorilla gorilla

Figure 2.5. Ankle joints of *H. sapiens, Au. afarensis, P. paniscus*, and *G. gorilla*. F, fibula, Tib, tibia, T, talus. The horizontal dotted line represents the horizontal axis of the tibiotalar joint. The continuous line joins the tips of the medial and lateral malleoli. In both *H. sapiens* and *Au. afarensis*, these two lines are approximately parallel. Latimer et al. [36] use this as evidence to predict that the *Au. afarensis* ankle joint would have enjoyed less mobility than that of the African apes. (Adapted with permission from Latimer B, Ohman JC, Lovejoy CO. Talocrural joint in African hominoids: implications for *Australopithecus afarensis*. Am J Phys Anthropol. 1987 Oct; 74(2):162. Copyright © 1987 John Wiley & Sons, Inc. Reprinted with permission of Wiley-Liss, Inc., a subsidiary of John Wiley & Sons, Inc.)

and Lovejoy [45] described this characteristic as intermediate between the African ape and the modern human conditions. In apes, the fibular trochlea has been interpreted as an adaptation for climbing. Both Stern and Susman [37] and Latimer and Lovejoy [45] suggest that the flat posterior calcaneal facet of *Au. afarensis* would have stabilised the talocalcaneal joint. Gebo [11] agrees this human-like flattening is present in the facet of the *Au. afarensis* calcaneum, but suggests that mobility at the joint was greater than that in modern humans because the facet extends proximally more than it does in modern humans. Another calcaneal trait found in *Au. afarensis* that Stern and Susman [37] associate with a plantigrade bipedal foot is a sustentaculum tali oriented perpendicular to the long axis of the calcaneum. However, Aiello and Dean [49] caution that the orientation of the sustentaculum tali does not differentiate modern humans and chimpanzees. At first, Stern and Susman [38] defined the broad body and calcaneal tuberosity of *Au. afarensis* as a bipedal feature. Later, they [79] refined their argument when they evaluated Latimer and Lovejoy's study [45]. Latimer and Lovejoy had plotted the cross-sectional widths of the calcaneal tuberosities of African apes, *Au. afarensis*, and humans. Their results showed the *Au. afarensis* values were within the human range. Stern and Susman added another *Au. afarensis* calcaneum Latimer and Lovejoy excluded on the basis of its poor condition, and the additional specimen fell within the gorilla range, and Stern and Susman suggest that this supports their argument that *Au. afarensis* was not exclusively bipedal.

Navicular: Clarke and Tobias [51] noted the humanlike *Au. afarensis* navicular tuberosity, but regarded the thin dorsal aspect of the navicular (the distance between the proximal articular for the talus and distal articular surface for the cuneiforms) and the pronounced angle between the facets for the intermediate and lateral cuneiform, as chimp-like traits. Interpretations vary as to the implications of navicular morphology with respect to whether *Au. afarensis* had a medial longitudinal arch. Stern and Susman [37] interpret the broad attachment sites for the cubonavicular and calcaneonavicular ligaments on the plantar region of the navicular as an indication of a medial longitudinal arch and of restricted mobility. In contrast, Sarmiento and Marcus [52] and Harcourt-Smith [53] suggest the large navicular tuberosity argues against the presence of a medial longitudinal arch. In addition Berillon [54] suggests that the apelike dorsal obliquity of the *Au. afarensis* navicular indicates a range of dorsiflexion that is inconsistent with a medial longitudinal arch.

Cuboid: Gebo [11] proposed that the primitive morphology of the fragmentary *Au. afarensis* cuboid [40] reflects a calcaneocuboid joint designed for apelike midtarsal flexion (i.e., a 'midtarsal break').

Cuneiforms: The convexity [37] and relative orientation [54] of the hallucial metatarsal facet on the medial cuneiform have been interpreted as apelike features. Latimer and Lovejoy [55] agree the distal articular surface of the medial cuneiform shows some convexity, but identify other traits that suggest the hallux of *Au. afarensis* was incapable of prehension. They interpret the orientation of the

Au. afarensis first tarsometatarsal joint, the presence of a mediolaterally-directed bony ridge on the joint surface, and the location of the groove for the tibialis anterior tendon, as modern human-like adaptations to stabilise the hallux. Susman and Stern [37] regard the proximodistal elongation of the lateral cuneiform as a modern human-like trait. Berillon [54] suggests that the medial side of the *Au. afarensis* foot is similar to African apes in its range of dorsiflexion.

Metatarsals: Susman and Stern [37,38] suggest the *Au. afarensis* first metatarsal is stout relative to the other metatarsals, but they view it as apelike with respect to its convex proximal articular surface and mediolaterally-rounded distal articular surface. In contrast, Latimer and Lovejoy [56] emphasise the modern human-like expansion of the dorsal and plantar region of the distal articular surface. Both Latimer and Lovejoy [56] and Stern and Susman [37] agree the inflated dorsal regions of the distal articular surfaces of the metatarsals are modern human-like in that they would have facilitated dorsiflexion at the metatarsophalangeal joints at toe-off. Latimer and Lovejoy [56] point out that *Au. afarensis* metatarsals lack the plantar inflation of the distal articular surfaces characteristic of African apes, and they suggest, *contra* Stern and Susman [37], this would have compromised its prehensile capabilities. Duncan et al. [29] found that comparing the distal articular surface of metatarsals among great apes (including humans) using Latimer and Lovejoy's methodology [56] fails to differentiate the taxa according to positional behaviour. The *Au. afarensis* fifth metatarsal is similar to that of the African apes with respect to the inclination of the dorsoplantar and mediolateral axes of the tarsometatarsal facet, and Berillon suggests these features are not compatible with a lateral longitudinal arch [54].

Phalanges: The phalanges of *Au. afarensis* are relatively long, slender, and curved like those of the great apes, and McHenry [57] noted the length of the intermediate fifth phalanx (AL333-115L) is outside the modern human range, but within the range of chimpanzees. Other apelike traits include plantar expansion of the shafts for the insertions of the flexor sheaths and the relative lengths of the second and third proximal phalanx [37]. In contrast, Latimer and Lovejoy's [56] ratios comparing phalangeal length to arm, pelvic, and leg lengths for both *Au. afarensis* and modern humans revealed similar proportions between these two groups. These results contrasted with Stern and Susman's [37] consideration of the ratio of phalangeal length and femoral head diameter in which *Au. afarensis* exceeds the modern human range.

Latimer and Lovejoy [56] suggest the orientation of the proximal articular surfaces of the *Au. afarensis* phalanges is modern human-like, but Duncan et al.'s [29] analysis determined that the orientation of the proximal articular surface of *Au. afarensis* phalanges was intermediate between those of the African apes and modern humans.

Footprints: Direct evidence of locomotion comes from the 3.8 to 3.4 Mya hominin footprint trails in the Laetoli Formation, at Laetoli, Tanzania (Figure 2.6).

The first footprints were recognised at Laetoli in 1976 and since then the tracks of more than 20 bird and mammal taxa have been recognised [58]. The prints were made in layers of volcanic ash called tuffs. The tuffs at Laetoli are particularly rich in a chemical called natrocarbonatite that dissolves in water to produce a carbonate-rich solution. This, when dried by the sun, cements the ash layer within a few hours. Researchers think that showers of ash fell in the dry season and that the animals must have walked across the wet ash soon after the beginning of the rainy season. Six layers preserve footprints, but most of the preserved prints are in two of them, and the hominin footprints are in one of these called the 'footprint tuff'. Trails of potential hominin prints have been excavated at two sites, A and G. The two trails, 1 and 2, at site G provide the best evidence and they preserve evidence of 22 and 12 prints, respectively. The number of individuals responsible for these two parallel trails is contested. Some researchers interpret the Site G trails as the footprints of three individuals, two individuals walking side by side followed by a third hominin directly behind one of the individuals [58,59]. Other researchers interpret the trails as the footprints of two individuals walking side by side [60,61].

Au. afarensis skeletal material at Laetoli is contemporaneous with the footprints, and this has led most researchers to link the trails with *Au. afarensis* [37,62–70]. A minority view, proposed by Tuttle and colleagues [59,71] is that

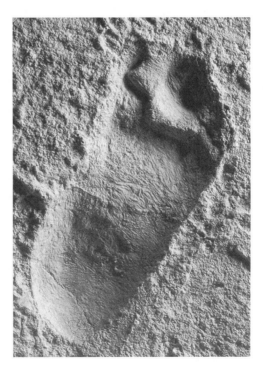

Figure 2.6. This footprint, part of a series of trackways found at Laetoli, Tanzania represents direct evidence that hominins were walking bipedally as early as 3.6 Mya. (Reprinted from Tatersall I, Schwartz J. Extinct Humans, page 89, Copyright 2000, Westview Press.)

Au. afarensis' long lateral digits would have resulted in footprints unlike those found at Laetoli, and they suggest the Laetoli footprints were made by another archaic hominin species that had feet more similar to those of modern humans. In response to Tuttle et al.'s claims, Schmid [72] explains that chimpanzees curl their long lateral toes and leave footprints hiding the true lengths of their lateral digits, a view supported by Stern and Susman [37]. White and Suwa's [70] reconstruction of the *Au. afarensis* foot is compatible with the Laetoli footprints, and they suggest that the apparent discrepancies between the prints and the foot fossils belonging to *Au. afarensis* may not be a result of toe-curling, but due to drag of the second toe on the substrate after toe-off.

Most researchers suggest the Laetoli footprints are evidence of a hominin with a fully adducted great toe [37,59,70,72], whereas others interpret them as evidence of a slightly or fully abducted hallux [61,73]. Several researchers [59,66,71,73,75] suggest the Laetoli footprints were made by a hominin with a medial longitudinal arche, but Stern and Susman [37] caution that a chimp footprint in sand can give the illusion of this feature. Meldrum [73] has noted that even though some Laetoli footprints appear to possess a medial longitudinal arch, they are not associated with pronounced impressions at the heel and first metatarsophalangeal joint – a notable feature of the modern human footprints even in volcanic ashlike substrate. Instead, Meldrum suggests the Laetoli footprints show a 'pressure ridge' (area associated with high plantar pressure in chimp feet) found in the navicular region [73], a lateral metatarsal area showing the greatest forefoot impressions [37,72,73], and a chimplike, tapering impression of the heel [73]. When Meldrum and Wunderlich [75] examined plantar pressures and kinematics in bipedal modern humans and chimpanzees, they found that flexion of the midtarsal region of the chimpanzee foot was associated with a Laetoli-like 'pressure ridge'. Flexion at the midtarsal region, the 'midtarsal break', allows the ape foot to comply with a vertical substrate during climbing. If this feature was present in the Laetoli hominins, it would suggest these individuals engaged in arboreal locomotion.

In another walking experiment Schmid [72] compared one group of individuals walking normally, with another group instructed to walk without swinging their arms. In this latter group the greatest forefoot pressure was on the head of the fifth metatarsal, the same location as the deepest part of the Laetoli forefoot impression. Schmid proposed that the funnel-shaped apelike thorax of *Au. afarensis* would not have allowed the type of arm swinging that efficiently balances the body during bipedalism.

Contrary to Meldrum and Wunderlich's [75] and Schmid's independent experimental studies [72] which provide support that Laetoli hominin feet lacked weight-bearing medial arches and would have exhibited more apelike gaits, other investigators propose the Laetoli hominins were fully upright striders [58,66,70,76]. After measuring velocity, stride length, and cadence, Charteris et al. [67,68] concluded the Laetoli Site G trackways are representative of a hominin with a modern human-like stroll. Although Tuttle et al. [59] disagree that assumptions of stature and speed prevent accuracy in assessing gait, they nonetheless support the prediction that Laetoli hominins had a modern humanlike stride.

Foot function and locomotion: Opinion about the locomotor regime of *Au. afarensis* is divided. Some researchers discount the primitive characteristics of the skeletal evidence and claim that *Au. afarensis* was an obligate biped [36,40,44,77,78]. Others give primitive and derived traits equal weight and suggest that *Au. afarensis* was capable of both arboreal and bipedal locomotion [37,38,79]. Some researchers suggest that differences in pedal morphology between larger and smaller individuals within the hypodigm indicate differences in locomotor strategy [37], whereas others suggest these are allometric differences within a common morphological and functional theme [36,80]. A third group of researchers agrees that two different locomotor patterns are present in the hypodigm, and interprets this as evidence that the hypodigm subsumes fossils from more than one taxon [81–84]. Senut et al. [23] identify the smaller, more arboreal, members of *Au. afarensis* as part of the lineage that eventually gave rise to the genus *Paranthropus*, and they suggest that the larger, more bipedal, *Au. afarensis* specimens belong to a separate taxon that is directly ancestral to the genus *Homo*.

Gait reconstruction: Inferences about the gait of *Au. afarensis* fall into three categories. One suggests that its posture and gait were indistinguishable from modern humans, the second suggests *Au. afarensis* used a 'bent hip, bent knee' chimpanzee-like posture during bipedal gait, and the third claims *Au. afarensis* used a bipedal gait that has no modern analogue [85]. Proponents of the first cite features of the foot [36], leg [86,87], and pelvis [86] of *Au. afarensis* as supporting evidence. Those who suggest *Au. afarensis* used a chimpanzee-like 'bent hip, bent knee' postural behaviour during bouts of bipedalism (Figure 2.7) cite different evidence and interpretations [39,38,88,89]. Other modeling studies have predicted that the energy costs of a 'bent hip, bent knee' posture and gait would have been higher than the costs of an upright posture [90–92]. In fact, Kramer and Eck's [92,94] model suggests that *Au. afarensis* would have expended less energy using a fully upright posture during walking than modern humans do, but more recent studies have cast doubt on these conclusions [93,95]. Others propose there are morphological reasons to question the 'bent hip, bent knee' hypothesis. Ward suggests that the wide, distally flattened, lateral femoral condyle is evidence of an extended knee [96], and that the large calcaneum [45] is evidence that the leg and foot were designed to support an upright biped. In addition, Latimer and Ward [97] suggest there is evidence of a lordosis in the lumbar part of the vertebral column of *Au. afarensis*. Taken together with the observation that a lumbar lordosis develops in Japanese macaques after they have been trained to adopt an upright bipedal gait [98–100], this evidence suggests that *Au. afarensis* did not use a 'bent hip, bent knee' gait.

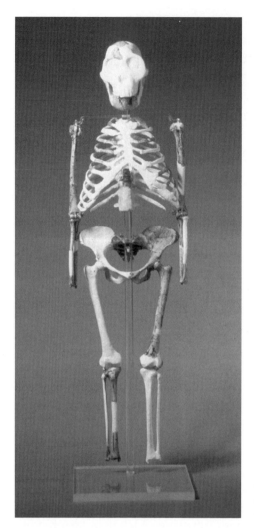

Figure 2.7. Reconstruction of 'Lucy' (AL-288-1), the 3.2 Mya partial Au. afarensis skeleton. Some scientists predict Au. afarensis would have exhibited a human-like stride, and others suggest that Lucy and her kind walked with a 'bent knee, bent hip', characteristic of occasional bipeds, such as chimpanzees. (Reproduced with permission from Peter Schmid.)

Summary: Assuming the skeletal evidence from Hadar and the trace fossil evidence from Laetoli represent one taxon, and if we weigh the primitive and derived characteristics observed in the Hadar pedal remains and in the Laetoli footprints, we conclude that the form and function of the *Au. afarensis* foot and thus the gait of *Au. afarensis* were not fully modern human-like. There is both experimental [72,73,75] and pedal skeletal evidence [37,38,47,52–54] that *Au. afarensis* most likely did not have a modern human-like longitudinal arch, and comparative analyses of the tibiotalar [36,39,38], talocalcaneal [11], talonavicular [40], calcaneocuboid [11], navicularcuneiform [54], and the first tarsometatarsal joint [37] all suggest that the *Au. afarensis* foot, compared to the modern human foot, enjoyed a greater range of motion. Furthermore, bone lengths in the foot of *Au. afarensis* argue for proportions that are closer to those found in chimpanzees [101] (Figure 2.8) and the long pedal phalanges may have affected gait [102].

Taxon name: Kenyanthropus platyops Leakey et al., 2001.

Approximate time range: ca. 3.5–3.3 Mya.

Source(s) of the evidence: West Turkana and perhaps Allia Bay, Kenya.

Nature of the evidence: The initial report lists the type cranium and the paratype maxilla plus 34 specimens (three mandible fragments, a maxilla fragment, and isolated teeth), some of which may also belong to the hypodigm, but at this stage the researchers are reserving their judgement about the taxonomy of many of these remains [103]. Some of them have only recently been referred to *Au. afarensis* [104].

Characteristics and inferred behaviour: The main reasons Leakey et al. [103] did not assign this material to *Au. afarensis* are its reduced subnasal prognathism, anteriorly-situated zygomatic root, flat and vertically-oriented malar region, relatively small but thick-enameled molars, and the unusually small M^1 compared to the size of the P^4 and M^3. Some of the morphology of the new genus including the shape of the face is *Paranthropus*-like yet it lacks the postcanine megadontia that characterises *Paranthropus*. The authors note the face of the new material resembles that of *Homo rudolfensis* (see below), but they rightly point out that the postcanine teeth of the latter are substantially larger than those of KNM-WT 40000. *K. platyops* apparently displays a hitherto unique combination of facial and dental morphology.

Pedal fossil evidence: None.

Taxon name: Australopithecus bahrelghazali, Brunet et al. [105].

Approximate time range: ca. 3.5–3.0 Mya.

Source(s) of the evidence: Koro Toro, Chad.

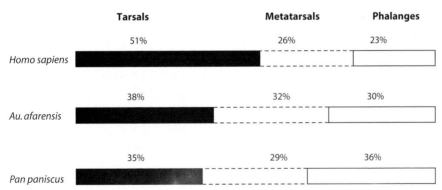

Figure 2.8. Foot proportions as indicated by lengths of tarsals, metatarsals, and phalanges of *H. sapiens, Au. afarensis*, and *P. paniscus*. Note that the proportions of *Au. afarensis* are similar to that of chimpanzees. The lack of complete distal phalanges in the *Au. afarensis* fossil assemblage indicates that toe lengths would have exceeded 30%. Stern [101] and Deloison [102] suggest that the long toes of these hominins would have been compatible with a foot adapted to arboreality, and would have given members a gait distinguishable from that of modern humans. (Adapted from Deloison Y. A new Hypothesis on the Origin of Hominid Locomotion, in Meldrum JD, Hilton CE. From Biped to Strider: The Emergence of Modern Human Walking, Running and Resource Transport, page 44, copyright 2004 Kluwer Academic Publishers Boston/Dordrecht London.)

Nature of the evidence: Published evidence is restricted to a fragment of the mandible and an isolated tooth.

Characteristics and inferred behaviour: Its discovers claim that its thicker enamel distinguishes the Chad remains from *Ar. ramidus* and that its smaller mandibular symphysis and more complex mandibular premolar roots distinguish it from *Au. afarensis*. Otherwise there is too little evidence to infer any behaviour.

Pedal fossil evidence: None.

Taxon name: Australopithecus africanus, Dart [106].

Approximate time range: ca. 3*–2.4 Mya.

Source(s) of the evidence: Most of the evidence comes from two caves, Sterkfontein and Makapansgat, with other evidence coming from Taung and Gladysvale.

Nature of the evidence: This is one of the best, if not the best, fossil record of an early hominin taxon. The cranium, mandible, and the dentition are well sampled. The postcranium and particularly the axial skeleton are less well represented in the sample, but there is at least one specimen of each of the long bones. However, many of the fossils have been crushed and deformed by rocks falling on the bones before they were fully fossilised.

Characteristics and inferred behaviour: Au. africanus had relatively large chewing teeth and apart from the reduced canines the skull is relatively apelike. Its mean endocranial volume, a reasonable proxy for brain size, is ca. 450 cm^3. The Sterkfontein evidence suggests that males and females of *Au. africanus* differed substantially in body size, but probably not to the degree they did in *Au. afarensis* (see above).

Pedal fossil evidence: Au. africanus is represented by two pedal assemblages. The older of the two is the partial left foot of StW 573 (Figure 2.9) that includes a talus, a fragmentary calcaneum, a navicular, three cuneiforms, and the proximal portion of the first metatarsal. The younger assemblage comprises a right calcaneum (StW 352), two right first metatarsals (StW 562, StW 595), a left second metatarsal (StW 377), two left third metatarsals (StW 477, StW 496), two right third metatarsals (StW 435, StW 388), a left (StW 485) and right (StW 596) fourth metatarsal, and a right fifth metatarsal (StW 114/115). It is possible that StW 377 and 485 belong to the same foot, with StW 388, 596, and 114/115 belonging to a second foot [101].

Talus: The *Au. africanus* talus shows a mosaic of ape and modern human affinities. The shape of the trochlear surface suggests that the ankle joint would have been more mobile than that of a modern human. However, other aspects of the

---

*N.B. It remains to be seen whether the associated skeleton StW 573 from Member 2 [51,60,107,108] and 12 hominin fossils recovered from the Jacovec Cavern since 1995 [109] belong to the *Au. africanus* hypodigm. Samples of quartz grains from Member 2 and the Jacovec Cavern have recently been dated to ca. 4.2–4.0 Mya [109].

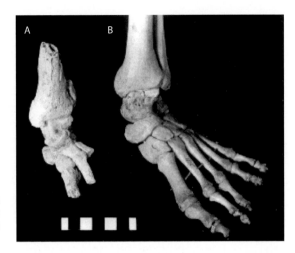

Figure 2.9. (A) StW 573 in comparison to its (B) modern human counterpart. Refer to text for description of the fossil. (Courtesy of Ron Clarke.)

shape of the trochlear and the vertical orientation of the groove for the flexor hallucis longus tendon [51,101] are modern humanlike features. Other characteristics shared with modern human tali are StW 573's short and stout body and the lack of anterior cupping of the medial malleolar facet [51]. Clarke and Tobias' measurements of the talar neck angle (the angle between the long axes of the trochlea and the talar neck) were in the human range [51], whereas Deloison [101] noted that the head is more expanded dorsally than ventrally, as it is in chimpanzee tali. Harcourt-Smith's [53] geometric morphometric analysis of the 3D shape of StW 573 also suggests that this talus is more apelike than modern humanlike.

Calcaneum: The calcaneocuboid facet of the fragmentary StW 573 calcaneum is chimpanzeelike, suggesting midtarsal mobility [101]. In contrast the younger calcaneum, StW 352, is more modern humanlike [101].

Navicular: The one notable humanlike characteristic of the StW 573 navicular is the form of its tuberosity [51], otherwise much of its preserved morphology, including the thin dorsal region where the cuneiforms articulate with the navicular, the large angle between the intermediate and lateral cuneiform facets and convex facets for the medial and intermediate cuneiforms [51,101], are apelike features. The overall shape of the navicular is intermediate between apes and modern humans [53].

Cuneiforms: The single, L-shaped facet on the medial cuneiform for the intermediate cuneiform is one trait StW 573 shares with modern humans [51,101]. Otherwise the tarsometatarsal articular surface of StW 573 shows more convexity and expansion onto the medial surface of the bone than in modern humans, and the well-developed articular surface for the second metatarsal, and the small bony prominence near the articular surface on its plantar aspect of the facet are apelike features [51,101]. Harcourt-Smith's analysis of the 3D shape of the medial cuneiform [53] has led him to conclude that the hallux was not abducted, whereas Clarke and Tobias [51] suggest the presence of facets for the fibularis longus tendon on both the medial cuneiform and first metatarsal indicate frequent opposition of the hallux. Deloison [101] describes the intermediate cuneiform as having an arboreally adapted tarsometatarsal joint. The lateral cuneiform possesses unique characteristics. The plantar region is more laterally directed than that of chimpanzees, and the facet for the navicular is smaller than in both chimpanzees and modern humans [101].

Metatarsals: Only the proximal portion of StW 573 is present. Its concave tarsometatarsal joint surface complements the convex facet on the medial cuneiform, suggesting a mobile first ray [51,101]. In the close-pack position (position at which the articular surfaces of a joint are maximally congruent), the angle of the first metatarsal [51] together with the strong bony impression for the fibularis longus tendon also suggests the hallux was abducted and capable of grasping [101]. The diaphyseal thickness of the first metatarsal is intermediate between that of chimpanzees and modern humans, and modern human first metatarsals are much less well developed laterally [101].

The StW 562 and StW 595 first metatarsals are similar to StW 573 in that their tarsometatarsal joint surface is concave [101]. The long axis of the shaft of StW 562 and StW 595 are both strongly curved, and other aspects of their morphology, including the distribution of bone around the distal articular surface is chimpanzeelike [101]. Deloison [101] describes the lateral metatarsals as exhibiting mixed morphologies of primitive and derived traits, but suggests that StW 496, 477, and 435 are adapted for bipedalism.

Foot function and locomotion: Opinions about the implications of the primitive and derived characteristics of the StW 573 foot are divided. Clarke and Tobias [51] conclude the talus is derived (i.e., modern humanlike), the navicular is intermediate between the modern human and ape condition, and the hallux was abducted and is therefore primitive. Harcourt-Smith and colleagues [53,110] present an alternative view. They also recognise that the navicular displays a mosaic of ape and modern human features, but they suggest that the talus is relatively apelike, and that the hallux was nonopposable. Despite the disagreement on which parts of the foot show greater or fewer primitive and derived characteristics, overall the pedal remains of *Au. africanus* suggest that this hominin could engage in both arboreal and bipedal locomotion [51,101]. This is consistent with conclusions reached by researchers who have studied other regions of the skeleton [85–87].

Megadont Archaic Hominins

This group includes hominin taxa conventionally included in the genus *Paranthropus* and one *Australopithecus* species, *Au. garhi.*

Taxon name: Paranthropus aethiopicus, Arambourg and Coppens [111,112] .

Approximate time range: ca. 2.5–2.3 Mya.

Source(s) of the evidence: Shungura Formation, Omo region, Ethiopia; West Turkana, Kenya.

Nature of the evidence: The hypodigm includes a well-preserved cranium from West Turkana (KNM-WT 17000), a few mandibles (e.g., KNM-WT 16005), and isolated teeth from the Shungura Formation. No postcranial fossils have been assigned to this taxon.

Characteristics and inferred behaviour: Similar to *P. boisei* (see below) except that the face is more prognathic, the cranial base is less flexed, the incisors are larger, and the postcanine teeth are not so large or derived. The only source of any endocranial volume data is KNM-ER WT17000. When this taxon was introduced in 1968 it was the only megadont hominin in this time range. With the discovery of *Au. garhi* (see below) it became apparent that robust mandibles with similar length premolar and molar tooth rows are being associated with what are claimed to be two distinct forms of cranial morphology.

Pedal fossil evidence: None.

Taxon name: Australopithecus garhi, Asfaw et al. [113].

Approximate time range: ca. 2.5 Mya.

Source(s) of the evidence: Bouri, Middle Awash, Ethiopia.

Nature of the evidence: A cranium and two partial mandibles.

Characteristics and inferred behaviour: Australopithecus garhi combines a primitive cranium with large-crowned postcanine teeth. However, unlike *Paranthropus* (see above) the incisors and canines are large and the enamel lacks the extreme thickness seen in the latter taxon. A partial skeleton combining a long femur with a long forearm was found nearby but is not associated with the type cranium of *Au. garhi* [113], but these fossils have not been formally assigned to *Au. garhi*.
Pedal fossil evidence: None.

Taxon name: Paranthropus boisei sensu stricto, Leakey [114,115].

Approximate time range: ca. 2.3–1.3 Mya.

Source(s) of the evidence: Olduvai and Peninj, Tanzania; Omo Shungura Formation and Konso, Ethiopia; Koobi Fora, Chesowanja, and West Turkana, Kenya; Melema, Malawi.

Nature of the evidence: P. boisei has a comprehensive craniodental fossil record. There are several skulls (the one from Konso being remarkably complete and well preserved), several well-preserved crania, and many mandibles and isolated teeth. There is evidence of both large and small-bodied individuals, and the range of the size difference suggests a substantial degree of sexual dimorphism. There are no cranial remains that can, with certainty, be assigned to *P. boisei*.

Characteristics and inferred behaviour: Paranthropus boisei is the only hominin to combine a massive, wide, flat face, massive premolars and molars, small anterior teeth, and a modest endocranial volume (ca. 450 cm^3). The face of *P. boisei* is larger and wider than that of *P. robustus,* yet their brain volumes are similar. The mandible of *P. boisei* has a larger and wider body or corpus than any other hominin (see *P. aethiopicus* above). The tooth crowns apparently grow at a faster rate than has been recorded for any other early hominin. There is, unfortunately, no postcranial evidence that can with certainty be attributed to *P. boisei.* The fossil record of *P. boisei* extends across about one million years of time during which there is little evidence of any substantial change in the size or shape of the components of the cranium, mandible, and dentition [116].

Pedal fossil evidence: None (but see the entry for *H. habilis sensu stricto*).

Taxon name: Paranthropus robustus, Broom [117].

Approximate time range: ca. 2.0--1.5 Mya.

Source(s) of the evidence: Kromdraai, Swartkrans, Gondolin, Drimolen, and Cooper's caves, all situated in, or near to, the Blauuwbank Valley, near Johannesburg, South Africa.

Nature of the evidence: The fossil record is similar to, but less numerous, than that of *Au. africanus.* The dentition is very well represented, some of the cranial remains are well preserved, but most of the mandibles are crushed and/or distorted. The postcranial skeleton is not well represented. Research at Drimolen was only initiated in 1992 yet already more than 80 hominin specimens have been recovered and it promises to be a rich source of evidence about *P. robustus.*

Characteristics and inferred behaviour: The brain, face, and chewing teeth of *P. robustus* are larger than those of *Au. africanus,* yet the incisor teeth are smaller. It has been suggested that the thumb of *P. robustus* would have been capable of the type of grip necessary for stone tool manufacture, but this claim is not accepted by all researchers.

Pedal fossil evidence:

Talus: The morphology of the trochlear of the TM 1517 talus from Kromdraai suggests a greater range of plantar flexion than in modern humans [11]. Several investigators [118–126] have suggested there is a functional relationship between the orientation of the neck of the talus and the degree of divergence of the hallux, but Lewis claims that torsion of the talar neck is only relevant to the orientation of the subtalar axis [35,127]. Day and Wood [124] found that whereas the horizontal talar neck angle of TM 1517 is intermediate between African apes and modern humans, the talar neck torsion angle (angle formed by the long axis of the anterior articular surface for the navicular and the trochlear plane) was closer to the modern human range. However, Robinson [128] interprets the morphology of TM 1517 as intermediate between that of a chimpanzee and a modern human, and suggested that its hallux was capable of opposition

[124,128,129]. Day and Wood measured the angle between the long axis of the neck of TM 1517 and the trochlear plane. This suggested that the medial part of the longitudinal arch was flatter than in modern humans [41,128].

Medial Cuneiform: The tarsometatarsal joint of the medial cuneiform (SKX 31117) is flat and is suggestive of an adducted hallux [79,130,131].

Metatarsals: The length of the first metatarsal (SKX 5017) is close to the female bonobo (pygmy chimpanzee) range. An ovoid-shaped proximal articular facet and a mediolaterally-wide plantar region of the distal articular facet are characteristics shared with chimpanzee metatarsals [133]. However, the flat superiorinferiorly-oriented proximal articular surface, the inferiorly-expanded basal region and proximal shaft indicating the presence of a plantar aponeurosis, the midshaft robusticity (diameter of the midpoint on the bone shaft relative to its length), and a distal articular surface that continues onto the dorsal region of the shaft are more modern humanlike features [79,131,132]. Other traits shared with modern humans are a mildly concave proximal articular surface and a prominent tubercle demarcating the insertion of the fibularis longus [79,131]. The angulation of the distal articular surface is more modern humanlike than chimpanzeelike [79,130]. A recently found first metatarsal from Swartkrans (SK 1813) also shares with SKX 5017 a mosaic of characteristics. The stratigraphic context and taxonomic status of this bone are unknown [135]. Susman and de Ruiter [135] noted both the humanlike and apelike characteristics of SK 1813. The humanlike traits include a large distal articular surface extending onto the dorsum of the bone, dorsoplantar expansion at the base, and an overall short, stout appearance. The apelike traits are a mediolaterally-narrow distal articular surface and axial rotation of the same articular surface. Susman and de Ruiter infer the humanlike traits of the metatarsal head would have allowed its owner to employ a dorsiflexed position at toe-off, but the apelike traits of the metatarsal head would have prevented close-packing at the metatarsophalangeal joint. A fifth metatarsal (SKX 33380) recovered from the same site displays humanlike characteristics such as a curved shaft and a bony crest marking the insertion where the fourth dorsal interosseus muscle attaches [131] (Figure 2.10).

Phalanges: Day and Thornton [136] concluded that the distal hallucial phalanx of *P. robustus* (TM 1517) is modern humanlike, particularly in its degree of axial torsion. Robinson [128] referred to a proximal phalanx, possibly belonging to the fifth digit, and a distal phalanx, belonging to either the second or third digit [128,137]. However, Musgrave [138] and Day [139] suggest that the distal phalanx is probably a hand and not a foot phalanx; and the proximal phalanx most likely belongs to a baboon [139]. The proximal hallucial phalanx (SK 45690) is modern humanlike in its shape and size [130,131] and the bony thickening on the basoplantar surface indicates the presence of a plantar aponeurosis [79]. A dorsally-canted proximal articular surface suggests humanlike dorsiflexion at the metarsophalangeal joint [79,131]. Furthermore, the presence of a prominent tubercle on the dorsal surface marks the attachment of extensor digitorum brevis [131].

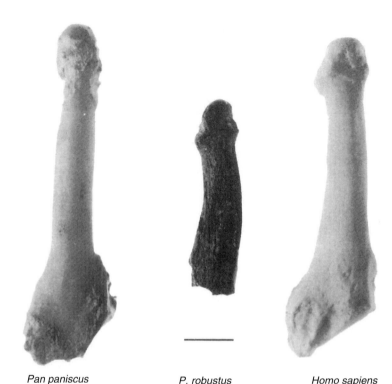

Pan paniscus   P. robustus   Homo sapiens

Figure 2.10.   The partial left fifth metatarsal of a P. robustus specimen, SKX 33380. It has a laterally curved shaft that is characteristic of a modern human. On the other hand, chimpanzee fifth metatarsals do not display this kind of diaphyseal attitude. This observation as well as other evidence from the pedal remains has led Susman [131] to conclude that P. robustus possessed a foot more similar to modern humans than to the African apes. (Image from Randall L. Susman, Stony Brook University, NY, USA in Brain CK. *Swartkrans: A Cave's Chronicle of Early Man,* page 130. © 1993 Transvaal Museum, Pretoria.)

Foot function and locomotion: Susman and Brain [132] suggest the SKX 5017 first metatarsal lacked grasping capabilities, but Susman and colleagues [79,132] also concluded that the weak markings for collateral ligaments indicate that *P. robustus* did not 'toe-off' at the hallux. Robinson [128] suggested the Kromdraai foot retained some arboreal capability, but Susman and Stern [79] cite the reduced finger curvature, more modern humanlike limb proportions, and the foot morphology as evidence that *P. robustus* was a more committed biped than, say, *Au. afarensis* or *Homo habilis* (see below). Napier [140] argued that if *P. robustus* was a biped then on the basis of its pelvic morphology it would have had a relatively inefficient system for weight transfer.

Archaic *Homo*

This group contains hominin taxa that are conventionally included within the *Homo* clade. Some researchers (e.g., [141]) have suggested that two of these taxa (*H. habilis sensu stricto* and *H. rudolfensis*) may not belong in the *Homo* clade, but until we have the means to generate sound phylogenetic hypotheses about these and other early hominin taxa it is not clear what their alternative generic attribution should be. Thus, for the purposes of this review these two taxa are retained within *Homo*.

Taxon name: Homo habilis sensu stricto, Leakey et al. [142].

Approximate time range: ca. 2.4–1.6 Mya.

Source(s) of the evidence: Olduvai Gorge, Tanzania; Koobi Fora and perhaps Chemeron, Kenya; Omo (Shungura) and Hadar, Ethiopia, East Africa; perhaps also Sterkfontein, Swartkrans, Cooper's, and Drimolen, South Africa.

Nature of the evidence: Mostly cranial and dental evidence with only a few post-cranial bones that can be confidently assigned to *H. habilis*.

Characteristics and inferred behaviour: The endocranial volume of *H. habilis* ranges from just less than 500 cm^3 to about 600 cm^3. All the crania are wider at the base than across the vault, but the face is broadest in its upper part. The curved proximal phalanges and well-developed muscle markings on the phalanges of OH 7 also indicate the hand was used for more powerful grasping (such as would be needed for arboreal activities) than is the case in any other species of *Homo*. The inference that *H. habilis* was capable of spoken language was based on links between endocranial morphology and, on the other hand, language comprehension and production that are no longer valid.

Pedal fossil evidence: The main pedal evidence for *H. habilis* is OH8[*] (but see the caveat in the section 'Foot function and locomotion' below). A partial subadult left foot (Figure 2.11) consisting of the talus, a portion of the calcaneum, the navicular, the cuboid, the three cuneiforms, and nearly complete metatarsals (1–5), has been attributed to *H. habilis*.

Talus: Lewis [35,127,143] suggests that the squat and foreshortened appearance of the OH 8 talus, together with the obliquely disposed subtalar and common anterior talocalcaneal facet orientations, the markings on the bones for the plantar flexor tendons, the lack of a medial head of flexor accessorius, and the form of the trochlear surface are chimpanzeelike features. The functional implications of the morphology of the head and neck of the talus has been interpreted differently by Day and Wood [124] and by Lisowski [122,123]. The former suggest the morphology is consistent with a longitudinal arch and an adducted hallux, whereas the latter suggests there is little or no evidence of a longitudinal arch, and interprets the hallux as being abducted. Kidd et al. [126] suggest that the torsion on the talar head is consistent with more mobility at the OH 8 talonavicular joint than would be usual in modern humans. The results of the multivariate analyses of Oxnard, Lisowski, and colleagues [126,144,145] suggest that OH8 and TM 1517, the *P. robustus* talus from Kromdraai, differ from both African ape and modern human tali, and most closely resemble the tali of the orangutan.

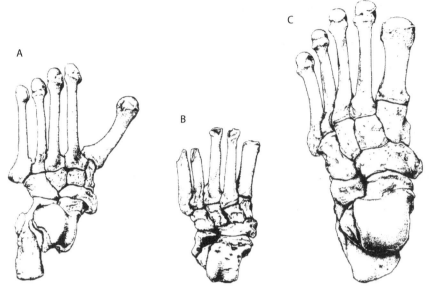

Figure 2.11. Tarsus and metatarsus of (A) a chimpanzee, (B) OH8, and (C) a modern human. OH8 is missing its calcaneal tuberele and the distal ends of its metatarsals. Based on their observations that the epiphysis of the second and third metatarsals had not completely fused, Susman and Stern [159] predict the foot belonged to a juvenile. (Reprinted with permission from the American College of Foot and Ankle Surgeons [74, p. 369].) Copyright © 1983 by the American Orthopedic Foot and Ankle Society (AOFAS), originally published in *Foot and Ankle International*, June 1983, Volume 3, Number 6, p. 369 and reproduced here with permission.

Calcaneum: Kidd et al. [126] and Berillon [54] argue that the morphology of the proximal calcaneum is consistent with a longitudinal arch [54,126].

Navicular: The tuberosity of the navicular is modern humanlike [125,146] and bony markings that are most likely for the cubonavicular and plantar calcaneonavicular ligaments are consistent with a longitudinal arch [52,146]. Sarmiento and Marcus [52] also cite the large, shallow talar facet and the orientations of the articular facets as further evidence of a longitudinal arch, but they suggest the latter was not as well developed as it is in modern humans. Athough Deloison suggests that the navicular is thicker dorsally than it is in the apes [101], Kidd et al.'s [126] multivariate analysis suggests morphological similarities between the navicular of OH8 and that of the apes.

Cuboid: The OH8 cuboid possesses a beak similar to that seen in modern humans; this acts to both restrict the range of motion in the calcaneocuboid joint [147] and support the lateral arch [148,149]. Lewis [150] noted that the beak is even more pronounced in OH8 than in modern humans and would have provided even more joint stability. In addition, Susman and Stern assert [38,146] that the OH8 calcaneocuboid joint is not consistent with a 'midtarsal break' during bipedal locomotion, and this is also the conclusion of a multivariate analysis of the OH8 cuboid [148]. Though Lewis [35,127,143] agrees the OH 8 cuboid resembles the form of the modern human cuboid, he suggests that movement between the cuboid and calcaneum would be more limited in the former.

Cuneiforms: The distal articular surface of the medial cuneiform is flat [38,101,146] and the facet does extend onto the medial surface [101], suggesting to some researchers that the hallux was not divergent. However, Lewis [35,127,143] concluded that OH 8 did have a divergent hallux. The intermediate cuneiform has been described by Harcourt-Smith and Aiello [152] as uniquely wedge-shaped, yet the rectangular lateral cuneiform [146] is said to be consistent with a modern humanlike transverse arch [11].

Metatarsals: The stout first metatarsal is in some ways modern humanlike [146]. Day and Napier [153] used the facet between the first and second metatarsal as evidence that the hallux was aligned with the rest of the foot, but Lewis [150] points out that this articulation may have been created by pseudoarthrosis. Lewis' [35,127,143] examination of the torsion of the first metatarsal led him to suggest the first ray may have possessed grasping capabilities. Susman and Stern's [146] observations differ from Lewis'. They described the hallucial metatarsal as exhibiting modern humanlike torsion and suggest that the hallux was not habitually abducted. Lewis [35,127,143] suggests that the second and third metatarsal morphology is a mosaic of modern human and apelike morphology. The fifth metatarsal is mediolaterally flat as in modern humans [146] and when robusticity (midpoint diameter divided by bone length) of the metatarsals has been compared across the foot, OH8 follows the modern human pattern [154].

Phalanges: The right terminal hallucial phalanx (OH10) has been described by Day and Napier [155] as exhibiting the uniquely human traits of lateral axial torsion (viewed from the distal end) and valgus deviation. The phalanx is also more broad than long, a characteristic shared with one of the two Neanderthal specimens in the comparative sample [155]. Because both *H. habilis* and *P. boisei* fossils have been found at Olduvai, Day and Napier did not assign this toe bone to a taxon. Later, Day's [156] multivariate analysis of OH10 argues for modern human affinities. In response, Oxnard [157] referred to the incongruence of the results of Day's canonical analysis and his own Mahalanobis distance values (D^2). In Oxnard's analysis [157] the 'D' values suggest that OH10 differs from both modern humans and African apes.

Foot function and locomotion: First, it should be made clear that there is no certainty that OH 8 and OH 10 belong to *H. habilis*; they could equally well belong to the other hominin known from Bed I at Olduvai, *P. boisei*. However, if we assume for the sake of argument that they are correctly assigned to *H. habilis*, then what can we conclude about the function of its foot?

There are differences of opinion about the position of the hallux, some investigators suggest it was adducted [38,101,124,146,153], others see evidence for full abduction [122,123,148], and a third group favours an intermediate position [35,52,143,151,158]. Likewise, there is disagreement about the likelihood that OH 8 had a longitudinal arch, with some researchers favouring the interpretation that it is modern human-like [38,54,153,159], others that it is completely absent [35,122,123,143,158], and a third group favouring an expression that is intermediate between apes and modern humans [52,124,148]. Elsewhere in the foot, there is evidence that the OH 8 foot is more flexible than it is in modern humans [127,143]. Overall, evidence from unambiguous *H. habilis* specimens such as OH 62 and OH 7 suggest that *H. habilis* was capable of traveling arboreally and bipedally [159]. However, the mosaic nature of the morphology of the OH 8 foot suggests that the bipedal gait of *H. habilis* differed from that of modern humans [35,124,126,143,152,158,160,161].

Taxon name: Homo ergaster Groves and Mazák, 1975.

Approximate time range: ca. 1.9–1.5 Mya.

Source(s) of the evidence: Koobi Fora, West Turkana, Kenya; Dmanisi, Georgia.

Nature of the evidence: Cranial, mandibular, and dental evidence, including a remarkably complete associated skeleton of a juvenile male individual from Nariokotome, West Turkana.

Characteristics and inferred behaviour: Two sets of features are claimed to distinguish *H. ergaster* from *H. erectus*. The first comprises features for which *H. ergaster* is more primitive than *H. erectus*, with the most compelling evidence coming from details of the mandibular premolars. The second set comprises features of the vault and base of the cranium for which *H. ergaster* is less specialised, or derived, than *H. erectus*. Overall *H. ergaster* is the first hominin to combine modern human-sized chewing teeth with a postcranial skeleton (e.g., long legs, large femoral head, etc.) apparently committed to long-range bipedalism and to lack morphological features associated with arboreal locomotor and postural behaviours. The small chewing teeth of *H. ergaster* imply that it was either eating different food than the australopiths, or that it was preparing the same food extraorally. This could have involved the use of stone tools, or cooking, or a combination of the two.

Pedal fossil evidence: The best source of evidence about the postcranial morphology of *H. ergaster* comes from associated skeletons, such as KNM-WT 15000 (Figure 2.12) and KNM-ER 1808 that include diagnostic cranial evidence. Unfortunately neither of these associated skeletons includes pedal fossils that are reliably linked to those specimens. The more fragmentary associated skeleton KNM-ER 803 which includes a talus, a left third metatarsal missing its distal articular surface, the base of a left fifth metatarsal, one proximal phalanx, two intermediate phalanges, a distal phalanx [163], and the KNM-ER 813 talus may well belong to *H. ergaster*, but they could equally well belong to *H. rudolfensis* (see below). Walker and Leakey [164] have identified a first metatarsal or metapodial fragment from the same stratigraphical context as the male subadult *H. ergaster* skeleton, KNM-WT 15000. Although this bone is consistent with the developmental morphology of KNM-WT 15000, some traits suggest it may instead belong to a young mammal. Presently, only a right third metatarsal (D2021) lacking its distal end has

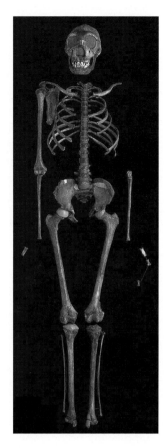

Figure 2.12. The juvenile skeleton KNM-WT 15000. *Homo ergaster* A metatarsal-like bone was found in the same layer as the skeleton, but it is not certain that it belongs with KNM-WT 15000. However, its human-like body proportions are much more modern-like than those of the australopiths, so it is very likely that *Homo ergaster* and *Homo erectus* were obligate bipeds. (Image kindly provided by National Museums of Kenya.)

been described from the Dmanisi site. Its size and proportions are similar to other hominin metatarsals, such as KNM-ER 15000, KNM-ER 803 and KNM-ER 1823, and D2021's shaft curvature and ventral basal tubercles are most comparable to KNM-ER 803 [165]. Its length suggest that it belonged to a small female [166]. The lateral facet of D2021 has a modern human-like ovoid shape, in contrast to the triangular shape exhibited by KNM-ER 803 [166]. Gabunia et al. [166] suggest the morphology of D2021 indicates it was part of a foot that had low longitudinal and transverse arches. Two intermediate phalanges belonging to KNM-ER 803 are short and straight compared to those belonging to *Au. afarensis* [44, 209].

Foot function and locomotion: Although debate surrounds the degree of relatedness between *H. ergaster* and *H. erectus* [167], it is generally agreed that both assemblages represent a grade which has surpassed archaic hominins and earlier *Homo* in terms of its ability to travel long distances efficiently [167,168]. Collectively, these changes in the hominin lineage with the appearance of modern human-like body [167 and references therein] suggest these hominins were habitual bipeds. KNM-WT15000 has limb proportions (long distal limb segments relative to corresponding proximal limb segments) that are most similar to modern Africans living in the tropics [169]. In order to test if KNM-WT15000's long tibial length relative to femoral length (associated with a high crural index) would have had any bearing on its gait, Gruss and Schmitt [170] compared the kinematics and kinetics of human subjects with high crural indices to those with lower crural indices. Gruss and Schmitt [170] found subjects with higher crural indices kept their knees more flexed throughout the stance phase to minimise forces on the hip. Also in the same subjects, the centre of pressure was found more anteriorly along the foot to provide more reinforcement against stress on the knee. It is possible that *H. ergaster* modified its posture in a similar fashion to keep ground reaction force to a minimum.

Taxon name: Homo rudolfensis, Alexeev [171] *sensu*, Wood [172].

Approximate time range: ca. 1.8–1.6 Mya.

Source(s) of the evidence: Koobi Fora, and perhaps Chemeron, Kenya; Uraha, Malawi.

Nature of the evidence: Several incomplete crania, two relatively well-preserved mandibles, and several isolated teeth.

Characteristics and inferred behaviour: Homo rudolfensis and *H. habilis* show different mixtures of primitive and derived features. For example, although the absolute size of the brain case is greater in *H. rudolfensis*, its face is widest in its midpart whereas the face of *H. habilis* is widest superiorly. Despite the absolute size of its brain (ca. 750–800cm^3) when it is related to estimates of body mass the brain of *H. rudolfensis* is not substantially larger than those of the australopiths. The more primitive face of *H. rudolfensis* is combined with a robust mandible and mandibular postcanine teeth with larger, broader, crowns and more complex premolar root systems than those of *H. habilis*. At present no postcranial remains can be reliably linked with *H. rudolfensis*. The mandible and postcanine teeth are larger than one would predict for a generalised hominoid of the same estimated body mass suggesting that its dietary niche made similar mechanical demands to those of the megadont australopiths.

Pedal fossil evidence: None (but see *H. ergaster*).

Taxon name: Homo erectus sensu stricto, Dubois [173] and Weidenreich [174].

Approximate time range: ca. 1.8 Mya–200 Kya.

Source(s) of the evidence: Sites in Java (e.g., Trinil, Sangiran, Sambungmachan), China (e.g., Zhoukoudian, Lantian), and Africa (e.g., Olduvai Gorge, Melka Kunture).

Nature of the evidence: Mainly cranial with some postcranial evidence, but little or no evidence of the hand or foot.

Characteristics and inferred behaviour: The crania belonging to *H. erectus* have a low vault, a substantial more-or-less continuous torus above the orbits, and the occipital region is sharply angulated. The inner and outer tables of the cranial vault are thick. The body of the mandible is less robust than that of the australopiths and in this respect it resembles *Homo sapiens* except that the symphyseal region lacks the well-marked chin that is a feature of later *Homo* and modern humans. The tooth crowns are generally larger and the premolar roots more complicated than those of modern humans. The cortical bone of the postcranial skeleton is thicker than is the case in modern humans. The limb bones are modern humanlike in their proportions and have robust shafts, but the shafts of the long bones of the lower limb are flattened from front to back (femur) and side to side (tibia) relative to those of modern humans. All the dental and cranial evidence points to a modern humanlike diet for *H. erectus* and the postcranial elements are consistent with a habitually upright posture and obligate, long-range bipedalism. There is no fossil evidence relevant to assessing the dexterity of *H. erectus*, but if *H. erectus* manufactured Acheulean artifacts then dexterity would be implicit.

Pedal fossil evidence: None.

Taxon name: Homo antecessor, Bermúdez de Castro et al. [175].

Approximate time range: ca. 700–500 Kya.

Source(s) of the evidence: Gran Dolina, Atapuerca, Spain.

Nature of the evidence: The partial cranium of a juvenile, parts of mandibles and maxillae, and isolated teeth.

Characteristics and inferred behaviour: Researchers who found the remains claim the combination of a modern humanlike facial morphology with the large and relatively primitive crowns and roots of the teeth is not seen in *H. heidelbergensis* (see below). The Gran Dolina remains show no sign of any derived *H. neanderthalensis* traits. Its discoverers suggest *H. antecessor* is the last common ancestor of Neanderthals and *H. sapiens*.

Pedal fossil evidence:

Metatarsals: The second metatarsal (ATD6-70+107) is similar to modern humans in overall morphology and dimensions. Its midshaft mediolateral diameter (midshaft breadth) relative to its midshaft dorsoplantar diameter (midshaft height), a measure of robusticity, is below the mean for either modern humans or Neanderthals [176].

Phalanges: Dimensions and robusticity indices of the hallucial proximal phalanges (ATD6-30 and ATD6-31) are comparable to those of modern humans, except that *H. antecessor* has longer phalanges relative to the shaft breadth. Overall, the *H. antecessor* phalanges are not as robust [0.5*(midshaft breadth + midshaft height)/articular length*100] as later fossil hominins from Sierra de Atapuerca (possible Neanderthal precursors), Neanderthals, and modern humans. However, the proximal rugosity index values (proximal articular surface height compared to proximal articular surface breadth) are similar among all the groups [176]. Lacking any association with a specific ray, the proximal phalanx (ATD6-32) was compared to phalanges from the second, third, and fourth ray of Neanderthals and modern humans [176]. Its midshaft breadth relative to midshaft height is intermediate between Neanderthals (upper range) and unshod and shod modern humans (lower range), but closest to early modern humans [176]. The middle phalanges (ATD6-33, ATD6-34, and ATD6-35) and the distal phalanges (ATD6-36 and ATD6-68) are not significantly different from those of the younger Sierra de Atapuerca hominins, Neanderthals, and modern humans.

Foot function and locomotion: The available fossil evidence suggests that the foot of *H. antecessor* functioned in much the same way as the modern human foot.

Taxon name: Homo heidelbergensis, Schoetensack [177].

Approximate time range: ca. 600–100 Kya.

Source(s) of the evidence: Sites in Europe (e.g., Mauer, Petralona), Near East (e.g., Zuttiyeh), Africa (e.g., Kabwe, Bodo), China (e.g., Dali, Jinniushan, Xujiayao, Yunxian), and possibly India (Hathnora).

Nature of the evidence: Many crania but little mandibular and postcranial evidence.

Characteristics and inferred behaviour: What sets this material apart from *H. sapiens* and *Homo neanderthalensis* (see below) is the morphology of the cranium and the robusticity of the postcranial skeleton. Some brain cases are as large as those of modern humans, but they are always more robustly built with a thickened occipital region and a projecting face, and with large separate ridges above the orbits unlike the more continuous brow ridge of *H. erectus*. Compared to *H. erectus* (see above) the parietals are expanded, the occipital is more rounded, and the frontal bone is broader. The crania of *H. heidelbergensis* lack the specialised features of *H. neanderthalensis* such as the anteriorly-projecting midface and the distinctive swelling of the occipital region. *H. heidelbergensis* is the earliest hominin to have a brain as large as anatomically-modern *H. sapiens* and its postcranial skeleton suggests that its robust long bones and large lower limb joints were well suited to long-distance bipedal walking.

Taxonomic note: Researchers who see distinctions between the African and non-African components of the hypodigm refer to the former as *Homo rhodesiensis*.

Pedal fossil evidence: One foot bone, a third metatarsal (Arago XLIII) from France, provides some information about the foot morphology of *H. heidelbergensis*. Overall, it is similar to metatarsals belonging to species of *Homo* including *H. sapiens*, but the shape of the metatarsal body is reminiscent of the morphology seen in OH 8 and the great apes. The Arago third metatarsal is more gracile than those belonging to Neanderthals [178].

Taxon name: Homo neanderthalensis, King [179].

Approximate time range: ca. >200–30 Kya.

Source(s) of the evidence: Fossil evidence for *H. neanderthalensis* has been found throughout Europe, with the exception of Scandinavia, as well as in the Near East, the Levant, and Western Asia.

Nature of the evidence: Many specimens are burials and so all anatomical regions are represented in the fossil record.

Characteristics and inferred behaviour: The distinctive features of the cranium of *H. neanderthalensis* include thick, double-arched brow ridges, a face that projects anteriorly in the midline, a large nose, laterally-projecting and rounded parietal bones, and a rounded, posteriorly-projecting occipital bone (i.e., an occipital 'bun'). The endocranial volume of *H. neanderthalensis* is, on average, larger than that of modern humans. Postcranially Neanderthals were stout with a broad rib cage, a long clavicle, a wide pelvis, and limb bones that are generally robust with well-developed muscle insertions. The distal extremities tend to be short compared to most modern *H. sapiens*, but Neanderthals were evidently obligate bipeds. The generally well-marked muscle attachments and the relative thickness of long bone shafts point to a strenuous lifestyle. The size and wear on the incisors suggest that the Neanderthals regularly used their anterior teeth as 'tools' either for food preparation or to grip hide or similar material.

Taxonomic note: The scope of the hypodigm of *H. neanderthalensis* depends on how inclusively the taxon is defined. For some researchers the taxon is restricted to fossils from Europe and the Near East that used to be referred to as 'Classic' Neanderthals. Others interpret the taxon more inclusively and include within the hypodigm fossil evidence that is generally older and less derived [e.g., Steinheim, Swanscombe, and Atapuerca (Sima de los Huesos)].

Recent developments: Researchers have recovered short fragments of mitochondrial DNA from the humerus of the Neanderthal type specimen [180,181]. The fossil sequence falls well outside the range of variation of a diverse sample of modern humans. Researchers suggest that Neanderthals would have been unlikely to have made any contribution to the modern human gene pool and they estimate this amount of difference points to 550–690 Kya of separation. Subsequently, mtDNA has been recovered at two other Neanderthal sites, from rib fragments of a child's skeleton recovered from Mezmaiskaya in the Caucasas [182] and from Vindija in Croatia [183]. Schmitz et al. [184] managed to extract mtDNA from the humeral shaft (NN 1) from a second individual at the Neanderthal type site. Serre et al. [185] extracted mtDNA from four more Neanderthal individuals, two more from Vindija (Vi 77 and 80), and from Engis 2 and La Chapelle-aux-Saints. The fragments of mtDNA that have been studied are short, but if the findings of the existing studies were to be repeated for other parts of the genome then the case for placing Neanderthals in a separate species from modern humans on the basis of their skeletal peculiarities would be greatly strengthened.

Pedal fossil evidence:

Talus: The neck angle, the talar neck torsional angle [122,124,186], and the differential height [122] of Neanderthal tali are comparable to those modern human tali. However, when multivariate methods are applied to these and other data the results are mixed. Some researchers conclude that Neanderthals are similar to modern humans [124], whereas others see some differences [157,187]. Rhoads and Trinkaus [186] found that the Neanderthal talus is taller, and the malleolar facets are more expanded. Squatting facets or facets caused by hyperdorsiflexion at the ankle are commonly found on both juvenile and adult Neanderthal skeletons (Figure 2.13). These facets are located on the anterior margin of the distal tibia, the dorsal area of the talar neck, the anterior medial malleolous, and the anterior trochlear [188]. Trinkaus [188] noted that the anterior and medial talar facets for the calcaneum are more often fused in modern human populations which are known to have engaged in habitual squatting, and this is also likely to have been the case in Neanderthals.

Calcaneum: The orientation and organisation of the sustentaculum tali are humanlike. The medial tuberosity, the attachment site for the calcaneal tendon, is larger than that in modern humans [189].

Overall tarsal morphology: Neanderthal and modern human tarsal articular facets are similar in relative size and orientation [189,190]. On the Neanderthal cuboid, the facet for the calcaneum is laterally expanded and is convex, indicating the presence of a lateral longitudinal arch and a stable midtarsal joint [189,190]. Like the calcaneum, the navicular and lateral cuneiform have larger tuberosites than found in modern humans [189].

Metatarsals: Early interpretations suggested the concave tarsometatarsal joints of Neanderthals meant that the first metatarsals were divergent [191–194]. However, Trinkaus [189] asserted that the Neanderthal first metatarsal was fully adducted and not twisted along its long axis to the same degree found in nonhuman primates. All Neanderthal metatarsals show the

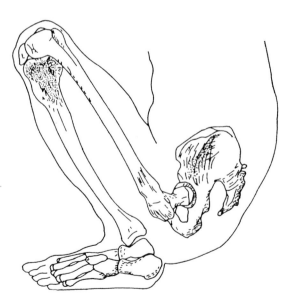

Figure 2.13. The presence of facets on the anterior border of the articular surface of the distal tibia and talus suggests Neanderthals habitually hyperdorsiflexed their feet, as one does while squatting for a prolonged period. (Reprinted from Trinkaus E. *Squatting among the Neandertals: a problem in the behavioral interpretation of skeletal morphology.* Journal of Archaeological Science, 1975;2:327–351, copyright 1975, with permission from Elsevier.)

same degree of torsion, basal orientation, and pattern of relative robusticity found in the human foot [190].

Phalanges: The Neanderthal proximal hallucial phalanx is within the normal range of valgus orientation characteristic of the modern human foot [189], but the hallucial proximal phalanx is more robust (midshaft breadth/shaft height) than those belonging to modern humans [195]. Neanderthal lateral (rays 2–4) proximal phalanges are more robust (greater mediolateral diaphyseal breadth relative to shaft length) and generally have more pronounced bony attachment sites for ligaments and tendons than those of modern humans [189]. Trinkaus and Hilton [195] suggest these features reflect greater locomotor demands on the Neanderthal foot compared to those on a modern human foot. The proximal hallucial phalanges (AT-96, AT-687, AT-772, AT-898, AT-899) from the Sima de los Huesos have a mean robusticity index that surpasses the means of *H. antecessor*, later Neanderthals, and modern humans [176].

Foot function and locomotion: When the Neanderthal foot bones are articulated in the close-pack position, they resemble a modern human-like foot with a longitudinal arch and inflexible tarsometatarsal [54,189]. Wedging of the intermediate and lateral cuneiforms, the orientation of the cuboid, and the medial rotation of the metatarsals' diaphyses also suggests that Neanderthals had a modern human-like transverse arch [161,189]. Attachment sites for plantar ligaments on the tarsals and metatarsals are also consistent with modern human-like arch structures [189].

Some key differences between Neanderthals and modern humans involve lower limb proportions. The medial subtalar length (the distance from the calcaneal tuberosity to the head of the first metatarsal) relative to the sum of the femoral and tibial lengths is somewhat greater in Neanderthals than in modern humans. In Neanderthals, the length of the rearfoot (calcaneal tuberosity to midtalar trochlea) compared to the anterior portion of the foot (midtalar trochlea to the distal articular surface of the first metatarsal) produces a ratio falling in the upper range for modern humans. Trinkaus [189] suggests this proportion is a result of the lengthening of the lever arm, thus increasing the mechanical advantage of the muscle attached to the calcaneal tendon. Furthermore, the proximal hallux length relative to the medial subtalar length reveals a smaller index than found in modern humans. In the few Neanderthal specimens with associated pedal phalanges that can be identified to ray, the intermediate and distal phalanges are relatively long compared to the associated proximal phalanx [189]. Trinkaus and Hilton [189,195] interpret these differences as suggesting that Neanderthal feet were subject to more stress, possibly due to locomotion over more rugged terrain. However, pronounced robusticity is not only found in the Neanderthal pedal skeleton, but is also seen throughout the skeletons of both juvenile and adult individuals [196,197].

Taxon name: Homo floresiensis, Brown et al. [198].

Approximate time range: ca. 95–18 Kya 2004.

Source(s) of the evidence: Only known from Liang Bua, a cave 500 m above sea level and 25 km from the north coast of Flores. The cave is in a limestone hill on the southern edge of the Wae Racang valley.

Nature of the evidence: A partial adult skeleton (LB1) with some components still articulated, an isolated left P$_3$ (LB2), and an unassociated left radius. The partial skeleton preserves the skull, and other components include the right pelvic bone, femur, and tibia.

Characteristics and inferred behaviour: This hominin (Figure 2.14) displays a unique combination of *Homo ergaster*-like cranial and dental morphology, a hitherto unknown suite of pelvic and femoral features, a small brain (ca. 380 cm^3), small body mass (25–30 kg), and small stature (1 m).

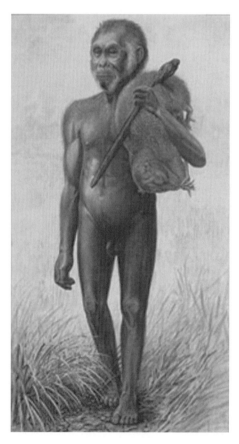

Figure 2.14. The Indonesian hominin assemblage attributed to *H. floresiensis* presents a mosaic of *H. ergaster* and modern humanlike traits. These bipeds only stood about 1 meter. Pedal remains have yet to be described. (Reprinted from Kemp M. Science in Culture. Nature 2004;432:555.)

Taxonomic note: The researchers responsible for the find decided, despite the small brain size, to nonetheless recognise its morphological affinities with *Homo* and include the new taxon within the genus *Homo*, but as a new species.

Pedal fossil evidence: No foot bones have been described.

Anatomically Modern *Homo*

Taxon name: Homo sapiens sensu stricto, Linnaeus [199].

Approximate time range: ca. 150 Kya to the present day.

Source(s) of the evidence: Fossil evidence of *H. sapiens s.s.* has been recovered from sites on all continents except Antarctica. The earliest absolutely dated remains are from Herto in Ethiopia [200] and from Omo Kibish [201].

Nature of the evidence: Many are burials so the fossil evidence is good, but in some regions of the world (e.g., West Africa) remains are few and far between.

Characteristics and inferred behaviour: The earliest evidence of anatomically-modern human morphology in the fossil record comes from sites in Africa and the Near East. It is also in Africa that there is evidence for a likely morphological precursor of anatomically-modern human morphology. This takes the form of crania that are generally more robust and archaic-looking than those of anatomically-modern humans yet which are not archaic enough to justify their allocation to *H. heidelbergensis* or derived enough to be *H. neanderthalensis* (see above). Specimens in this category include Jebel Irhoud from North Africa, Omo 2 and Laetoli 18 from East Africa, and Florisbad and Cave of Hearths in southern Africa. There is undoubtedly a gradation in morphology that makes it difficult to set the boundary between anatomically-modern humans and *H. heidelbergensis*, but unless at least one other taxon is recognized, the variation in the later *Homo* fossil record is too great to be accommodated in a single taxon.

Taxonomic note: Researchers who wish to make a taxonomic distinction between fossils such as Florisbad, Omo 2, and Laetoli 18 and subrecent and living modern humans refer the African subset to *Homo helmei* [202].

Pedal fossil evidence: The earliest pedal fossils assigned to *Homo sapiens* are from the Middle Eastern site of Skhul [190], the Ethiopian site of the Omo (Kibish) [203,204], and from Klasies River Mouth [205] .

Foot function and locomotion: The Skhul hominin pedal remains are in many respects functionally indistinguishable from those of modern humans. They have similar foot to leg proportions, proximal phalangeal relative lengths, and the phalanges show similar degrees of tendon and ligament bony markings [190]. However, the Skhul proximal pedal phalanges are intermediate between Neanderthals and later modern humans in shaft robusticity (mediolateral breadth relative to bone length), suggesting that modern humans made less demands on their forefoot over time [195]. The Skhul hominins also share some features with Neanderthals that are not seen in modern humans. These include a proximodistally short talar body relative to its height, a higher robusticity index for the first metatarsal [(dorsoplantar diameter + midshaft mediolateral diameter)/bone length], and slightly longer posterior pedal moment arm (distance between the middle region of the medial trochlea to the posterior edge of the calcaneal tuberosity) [190].

The first metatarsal belonging to the partial skeleton (Omo 1) of an anatomically-modern human from the Ethiopian site known as Omo (Kibish) and first metatarsal from the site of Klasies River Mouth which are both likely to date from more than 100 Kya are described as being indistinguishable from that of a modern human [204]. On balance, it is reasonable to conclude that the locomotion of the early members of *Homo sapiens* was indistinguishable from the locomotion of living modern humans.

Summary

So, how old are our feet? Feet, not necessarily like modern human feet, are more than 350 million years old. These early tetrapod feet had digits and tarsal bones, but they were at the end of hindlimbs that were splayed out laterally, not placed beneath the trunk. Their tarsal bones were more numerous and more homogeneous in appearance than modern human tarsal bones, but by 300 million years ago our reptilian ancestors had evolved two proximal tarsal bones that are recognisable as a calcaneum and a talus. A recognisable ankle joint, and the navicular, cuboid, and cuneiforms do not make their appearance until about 225 million years ago with the emergence of the primitive mammals.

Our more recent (between 65–55 million years ago) ancestors, the primitive primates, unlike many other mammalian groups, had very generalised feet, retaining all five metatarsals and five functional digits. This contrasts with other mammals like the ungulates that retain either just one (e.g., horses), or two (e.g., sheep), metatarsals. We are descended from Old World primates that have lost 'extra' bones such as the prehallux, although some of these 'lost' bones can turn up in otherwise normal individuals, and they can be confused with fractures unless the radiologist is experienced and knows something about evolutionary history and is thus aware of the potential for 'extra' bones in the feet.

Predators and scavengers have such a liking for the red marrow in the tarsal bones that they usually consume the feet, making them relatively rare as fossils. Thus, the fossil record of the foot is very sketchy until our ancestors started to deliberately bury their dead and thus protect corpses from scavengers. Despite this sparse fossil record we are confident that our ancestors had grasping type feet until around two million years ago. The first evidence of a foot that resembles the feet of modern humans appears in the fossil record just less than two million years ago, but by this time it is likely that most of the distinctive elements of our feet were present. These include a short compact talus, modest but definite longitudinal and transverse arches, and midfoot joints that 'lock' to convert the tarsus into a stiff lever that can transmit the force generated by the calf muscles to the hallux to produce a powerful 'toe-off'.

Thus, compared to the elbow, or hip joint, our feet are relatively recently evolved structures. Likewise, our dependency on our feet for support and propulsion is also relatively recent. This may explain why our feet are one of the parts of our body, like our backs and the veins of our lower limbs, that are prone to show signs of maladaptation and malfunction.

References

1. Wildman D, Grossman LI, Goodman M. Functional DNA in humans and chimpanzees shows they are more similar to each other than either is to other apes. In: Moffat AS, ed. *Probing Human Origins*, Cambridge: American Academy of Arts and Sciences; 2002: 1–10.
2. Caccone A, Powell JR. DNA divergence among hominoids. *Evolution*, 1989; 43: 925–942.
3. Bailey WJ, et al. Reexamination of the African hominoid trichotomy with additional sequences from the primate beta-globin gene. *Molec Phylogen Evol*. 1992; 1: 97–135.
4. Horai S, et al. Recent African origin of modern humans revealed by complete sequences of hominoid mitochondrial DNAs. *Proc Nat Acad Sci USA*. 1995; 92: 532–536.
5. Gagneux P, Woodruff DS, Boesch C. Retraction: Furtive mating in female chimpanzees. *Nature*. 2001; 414: 508.
6. Wildman D, et al. Implications of natural selection in shaping 99.4% nonsynonymous DNA identity between humans and chimpanzees: Enlarging genus *Homo*. *Proc Nat Acad Sci*. 2003; 100: 7181–7188.
7. Shi J, et al. Divergence of the genes on human chromosome 21 between human and other hominoids and variation of substitution rates among transcription units. *Proc Nat Acad Sci*. 2003; 100: 8331–8336.
8. Arnason U, Janke A. Mitogenomic analyses of eutherian relationships. *Cytogenetic Genome Res*. 2002; 96: 20–32.
9. Huxley JS. Evolutionary process and taxonomy with special reference to grades. *Upps Univ Arssks*. 1958: 21–38.
10. Ruvolo M. Genetic diversity in hominoid primates. *Ann Rev Anthrop*. 1997; 26: 515–540.
11. Gebo DL. Plantigrady and foot adaptation in African apes: Implications for hominid origins. *Am J Phys Anthrop*. 1992; 89: 29–58.
12. Rose MD. The process of bipedalization in hominids. In: Senut B, ed. *Origine(s) de la Bipédie Chez les Hominidés*. Paris: CNRS; 1991: 37–48.
13. Wheeler PE. The thermoregulatory advantages of hominid bipedalism in open equatorial environments: The contribution of increased convective heat loss and cutaneous evaporative cooling. *J Human Evol*. 1991; 21: 107–115.
14. Kortlandt A. How might early hominids have defended themselves against large predators and food competitors? *J Human Evol*. 1980; 9: 79–112.
15. Jablonski NG, Chaplin G. Origin of terrestrial bipedalism in the ancestor of the Hominidae. *J Human Evol*. 1993; 24: 259–280.

16. Hunt KD. The evolution of human bipedality: Ecology and functional morphology. *J Human Evol*. 1994; 26: 183–202.
17. Carrier DR. The energetic paradox of human running and hominid evolution. *Current Anthrop*. 1984; 25: 483–495.
18. Bramble DM, Lieberman DE. Endurance running and the evolution of *Homo*. *Nature*. 2004; 432: 345–352.
19. Wood, BA. Richmond BG. Human evolution: Taxonomy and paleobiology. *J Anat*. 2000; 196: 19–60.
20. Hartwig WC. ed. *The Primate Fossil Record*. Cambridge: Cambridge University Press; 2002:1–530.
21. Wood B, Constantino P. Human origins: Life at the top of the tree. In: Donoghue MJ, ed. *Assembling the Tree of Life*. New York: Oxford University Press; 2004: 517–535.
22. Brunet M, et al. A new hominid from the Upper Miocene of Chad, Central Africa. *Nature*. 2002; 145: 145–151.
23. Senut B, et al. First hominid from the Miocene (Lukeino formation, Kenya). *CR Acad Sci.-Series IIA-Earth Planetary Sci*. 2001; 332:137–144.
24. Pickford M, et al. Bipedalism in *Orrorin tugenensis* revealed by its femora. *CR Palevo.*, 2002; 1: 1–13.
25. Galick K, et al. External and internal morphology of the BAR 1002′ 00 *Orrorin tugenensis* femur. *Science*, 2004: 1450–1453.
26. Haile-Selassie Y, Asfaw B, White TD. Hominid cranial remains from Upper Pleistocene deposits at Aduma, Middle Awash, Ethiopia. *Am J Phys Anthrop*. 2004. 123:1–10.
27. Haile-Selassie, Y. Late Miocene hominids from the Middle Awash, Ethiopia. *Nature*. 2001; 412: 178–181.
28. Richmond BG, Begun DR, Strait DS. Origin of human bipedalism: The knuckle-walking hypothesis revisited. *Am J Phys Anthrop*. 2001; *Yrbk Phys Anthrop*. 44: 70–105.
29. Duncan A, Kappelman J, Shapiro L. Metatarsophalangeal joint function and positional behavior in *Australopithecus afarensis*. *Am J Phys Anthrop*. 1994; 93: 67–81.
30. White TD, Suwa G, Asfaw B. *Australopithecus ramidus,* a new species of early hominid from Aramis, Ethiopia. *Nature*. 1994; 371: 306–312.
31. White, TD, Suwa G, Asfaw B. *Australopithecus ramidus,* a new species of early hominid from Aramis, Ethiopia -A corrigendum. *Nature*. 1995; 375: 88.
32. Semaw S, et al. Early Pliocene hominids from Gona, Ethiopia. *Nature*. 2005; 433: 301–305.
33. Leakey MG, et al. New four-million-year-old hominid species from Kanapoi and Allia Bay, Kenya. *Nature*. 1995; 376: 565–571.
34. Johanson DC, White TD, Coppens Y. A new species of the genus *Australopithecus* (Primates: Hominidae) from the Pliocene of East Africa. *Kirtlandia*. 1978; 28:1–14.
35. Lewis OJ. *Functional Morphology of the Evolving Hand and Foot*. Oxford: Oxford University Press; 1989.
36. Latimer B, Ohman J, Lovejoy C. Talocrural joint in African hominoids: Implications for *Australopithecus afarensis*. *Am J Phys Anthrop*. 1987; 74: 155–175.
37. Stern J, Susman R. The locomotor anatomy of *Australopithecus afarensis*. *Am J Phys Anthrop*. 1983; 60: 279–317.
38. Susman RL. Evolution of the human foot: Evidence from Plio-Pleistocene hominids. *Foot and Ankle*. 1983; 3: 365–376.
39. Susman R, Stern J, Jungers W. Arboreality and bipedality in the Hadar hominids. *Folia Primatol*. 1984; 43: 113–156.
40. Gomberg D, Latimer B. Observations on the transverse tarsal joint of *A. afarensis*, and some comments on the interpretation of behavior from morphology. *Am J Phys Anthrop Supplement*. 1984; 63:164.

41. Lamy P. The settlement of the longitudinal plantar arch of some African Plio-Pleistocene hominids: A morphological study. *J Hum Evol.* 1986; 15: 31–46.

42. Langdon J, Bruckner J, Baker H. Pedal mechanics and bipedalism in early hominids. In: Coppens Y, ed. *In Origine(s) de lat Bipédie Chez les Homindés*, Paris: CNRS; 1991:159–167.

43. Weidenreich F. Ueber die Beziehungen zwischen Muskelapparat und Knochen und den Charakter des Knochengewebes. *Ver Anat Ges Erlangen.* 1922: 28–53.

44. Latimer B, et al. Hominid tarsal, metatarsal and phalangeal bones recovered from the Hadar Formation: 1974–1977 collections. *Am J Phys Anthrop.* 1982: 74: 155–175.

45. Latimer B, Lovejoy C. The calcaneus of *Australopithecus afarensis* and its implications for the evolution of bipedality. *Am J Phys Anthrop.* 1989; 78: 369–386.

46. Weaver KF. The search for our ancestors. *Nat Geographic.* 1985: 566.

47. Deloison Y. Comparative study of calcanei of primates and *Pan-Australopithecus-Homo* relationship. In: Tobias PV, ed. *Hominid Evolution: Past, Present and Future.* New York: Alan R. Liss; 1985: 143–147.

48. Lewis OJ. The evolutionary emergence and refinement of the mammalian pattern of foot architecture. *J Anat.* 1983; 137: 21–45.

49. Aiello L, Dean C. *An Introduction to Human Evolutionary Anatomy.* London: Academic; 2001.

50. Susman RL. Species attribution of the Swartkrans thumb metacarpals: Reply to Drs. Trinkaus and Long. *Am J Phys Anthrop.* 1991; 86: 549–552.

51. Clarke R, Tobias P. Sterkfontein member 2 foot bones of the oldest South African hominid. *Science.* 1995; 269: 521–524.

52. Sarmiento EE, Marcus LF. The os navicular of humans, great apes, OH 8, Hadar, and *Oreopithecus*: Function, phylogeny, and multivariate analyses. *Am Museum Novitates.* 2000; 3288: 1–38.

53. Harcourt-Smith W. *Form and Function in the Hominoid Tarsal Skeleton.* London: University College London; 2002.

54. Berillon, G., In what manner did they walk on two legs? An architectural perspective for the functional diagnostics of the early hominid foot. In: Hilton C, ed. *From Biped to Strider: The Emergence of Modern Human Walking, Running, and Resource Transport.* New York: Kluwer Academic/Plenum; 2004.

55. Latimer B, Lovejoy C. Hallucal tarsometatarsal joint in *Australopithecus afarensis. Am J Phys Anthrop.* 1990a; 82: 125–133.

56. Latimer B, Lovejoy C. Metatarsophalangeal joints of *Australopithecus afarensis.* Am J Phys Anthrop. 1990b; 83: 13–23.

57. McHenry, HM. The first bipeds: A comparison of the *A. afarensis* and *A. africanus postcranium* and *implications* for the evolution of bipedalism. *J Human Evol.* 1986; 15: 177–191.

58. Leakey M, Hay R. Pliocene footprints in the Laetoli beds at Laetoli, North Tanzania. *Nature.* 1979; 278: 317–323.

59. Tuttle R, Webb D, Tuttle N. Laetoli footprint trails and the evolution of hominid bipedalism. In: Senut B, ed. *Origine(s) de la Bipédie chez les Homindés.* Paris: CNRS; 1991: 187–198.

60. Clarke RJ. Discovery of complete arm and hand of the 3.3 million-year-old *Australopithecus* skeleton from Sterkfontein. *S African J Sci.* 1999; 95: 477–480.

61. Deloison Y. Did Australopithecines walk as we do? In: Senut B, ed. *Origine(s) de la Bipédie chez les Homindés.* Paris: CNRS; 1991: 177–185.

62. Clarke R. Early hominid footprints from Tanzania. *S African J Sci.* 1979; 75: 148–149.

63. Johanson DC, White TD. A systematic assessment of early African hominids. *Science.* 1979; 202: 321–330.

64. Kemp M. Science in culture. *Nature.* 2004; 432: 555.

65. Day MH, Wickens EH. Laetoli Pliocene hominid footprints and bipedalism. *Nature.* 1980; 286: 385–387.

66. White TD. Evolutionary implications of Pliocene hominid footprints. *Science*. 1980; 208: 175–176.
67. Charteris J, Wall JC, Nottrodt JW. Functional reconstruction of gait from the Pliocene hominid footprints at Laetoli, northern Tanzania. *Nature*. 1981; 290: 496–498.
68. Charteris, J, Wall, JC, Nottrodt, JW. Pliocene hominid gait: New interpretations based on available footprint data from Laetoli. *Am J Phys Anthrop*. 1982; 58: 133–144.
69. Robbins L. Hominid footprints from site G. In: Harris J, ed. *Laetoli: A Pliocene Site in Northern Tanzania*. Oxford: Oxford University Press; 1987: 497–502.
70. White T, Suwa G. Hominid footprints at Laetoli: Facts and interpretations. Am J Phys Anthrop. 1987; 72: 485–514.
71. Tuttle RH. Ape footprints and Laetoli impressions: A response to the SUNY claims. In: Tobias PV, ed. *Hominid Evolution: Past, Present and Future*, New York: Alan R. Liss; 1985:129–133.
72. Schmid P. Functional interpretation of the Laetoli footprints. In: Hilton C, ed. *From Biped to Strider: The Emergence of Modern Human Walking, Running, and Resource Transport*. New York: Kluwer Academic/Plenum; 2004: 49–62.
73. Meldrum D. Fossilized Hawaiian footprints compared with Laetoli hominid footprints. In: Hilton C, ed. *From Biped to Strider: The Emergence of Modern Human Walking, Running, and Resource Transport*. New York: Kluwer Academic/Plenum; 2004: 63–83.
74. Susman RL. Evolution of the human foot: evidence from Plio-Pleistocene hominids. *Foot Ankle Int*. 1983; 3: 365-376.
75. Meldrum D, Wunderlich R. Midtarsal flexibility in ape foot dynamics, early hominid footprints and bipedalism. *Am J Phys Anthrop Supplement*. 1998; 26: 161.
76. Leakey MD. Tracks and tools. *Phil Trans R Soc London Ser B*. 1981; 292: 95–102.
77. Johanson DC, et al. Morphology of the Pliocene partial hominid skeleton (AL288-1) from the Hadar Formation, Ethiopia. *Am J Phys Anthrop*. 1982; 57: 403–451.
78. Latimer BM. Locomotor adaptations in *Australopithecus afarensis*: The issue of arboreality. In: Senut B, ed. *Origine(s) de la Bipédie chez les Hominidés*. Paris: CNRS; 1991:169–176.
79. Susman RL, Stern JT. Locomotor behavior of early hominids: Epistemology and fossil evidence. In: Senut B, ed. *Origine(s) de la Bipédie Chez les Hominidés*, Paris: CNRS;1991:121–131.
80. Ward CV, et al. South Turkwel: A new Pliocene hominid site in Kenya. *J Human Evol*.1999; 36: 69–95.
81. Deloison Y. L'Homme ne descend pas d'un primate arboricole! uné evidence méconnue. *Biom Hum et Anthropol*. 1999; 17: 147–150.
82. Senut B, Tardieu C. Functional aspects of Plio-Pleistocene hominid limb bones: Implications for taxonomy and phylogeny. In: Delson E, ed. *Ancestors: The Hard Evidence*. New York: Alan R. Liss; 1985: 193–201.
83. Tardieu C. *Analyse morpho-functionelle de l'articulation du genou chez les primates. Application aux hominides fossiles*. Paris: Universite of Pierre et Marie Curie; 1979.
84. Tardieu C. Morpho-functional analysis of the articular surfaces of the knee-joint in primates. In: Corruccini RS, ed. *Primate Evolutionary Biology*. Berlin: Springer-Verlag; 1981: 68–80.
85. Rak Y. Lucy's pelvic anatomy: Its role in bipedal gait. *J Human Evol*. 1991; 20: 283–291.
86. Lovejoy CO. Evolution of human walking. *Sci Am*. 1988; 259: 118–125.
87. Lovejoy CO, et al. The Maka femur and its bearing on the antiquity of human walking: Applying contemporary concepts of morphogenesis to the human fossil record. *Am J Phys Anthrop*. 2002; 119: 97–133.
88. Preuschoft H, Witte H. Biomechanical reasons for the evolution of hominid body shape. In: Coppens Y, ed. *Origine(s) de la Bipédie chez les Hominidés*. Paris: CNRS; 1991: 59–77.
89. Stern JT. The cost of bent-knee, bent-hip bipedal gait. A reply to Crompton et al. *J Human Evol*. 1999; 36: 567–570.
90. Ishida H. A strategy for long distance walking in the earliest hominids: Effect of posture on energy expenditure during bipedal walking. In: Senut B, ed. *Origine(s) de la Bipédie chez les Hominidés*. Paris: CNRS; 1991: 9–15.

91. Crompton RH, et al. The mechanical effectiveness of erect and "bent-hip, bent-knee" bipedal walking in *Australopithecus afarensis. J Human Evol*. 1998; 35: 55–74.
92. Kramer P, Eck G. Locomotor energetics and leg length in hominid bipedality. *J Human Evol*. 2000; 38: 651–666.
93. Nagano A, et al. Neuromusculoskeletal computer modeling and simulation of upright, straight-legged, bipedal locomotion of *Australopithecus afarensis* (A.L. 288-1). *Am J Phys Anthrop*. 2005; 126: 2–13.
94. Kramer PA. Modelling the locomotor energetics of extinct hominids. *J Exper Biol*. 1999; 202: 2807–2818.
95. Wang W, et al. Energy transformation during erect and 'bent-hip, bent-knee' walking by humans with implications for the evolution of bipedalism. *J Human Evol*. 2003; 44: 563–579.
96. Ward CV. Interpreting the posture and locomotion of *Australopithecus afarensis*: where do we stand? Phys. Anthrop. 2002; 45:185-215.
97. Latimer B, Ward CV. The thoracic and lumbar vertebrae. In: Leakey R, ed. *The Nariokotome* Homo erectus *Skeleton*, Cambridge, MA: Harvard University Press; 1993: 266–293.
98. Hayama S. Spinal compensatory curvature found in Japanese macaques trained for the acquisition of bipedalism. *Growth*. 1986; 35: 161–178.
99. Preuschoft H, Hayama S, Günther M. Curvature of the lumbar spine as a consequence of mechanical necessities in Japanese macaques trained for bipedalism. *Folia Primat*. 1988; 50: 42–58.
100. Nakatsukasa M. Acquisition of bipedalism: The Miocene hominoid record and modern analogues for bipedal protohominids. *J Anat*. 2004; 204: 385–402.
101. Stern JT. Climbing to the top: A personal memoir of *Australopithecus afarensis*. Evol Anthrop. 2000; 9:113–133.
102. Deloison Y. A new hypothesis on the origin of hominoid locomotion. In: Hilton C, ed. *From Biped to Strider: The Emergence of Modern Human Walking, Running, and Resource Transport* New York: Kluwer Academic/Plenum; 2004: 35–47.
103. Leakey MG, et al. New hominin genus from eastern Africa shows diverse middle Pliocene lineages. *Nature*. 2001; 410: 433–440.
104. Brown B, Brown FH, Walker A. New hominids from the Lake Turkana Basin, Kenya. *J Human Evol*. 2001; 41: 29–44.
105. Brunet M, et al. *Australopithecus bahrelghazli*, une nouvelle espece d'Hominide ancien de la region de Koro Toro (Tchad). *Comptes rendus de l'Academie des sciences*. 1996; 322: 907–913.
106. Dart R. *Australopithecus africanus,* the man-ape of South Africa. *Nature*. 1925; 115: 195–199.
107. Clarke RJ. First ever discovery of a well-preserved skull and associated skeleton of *Australopithecus*. *South African J Sci*.1998; 94: 460–463.
108. Clarke RJ. Newly revealed information on the Sterkfontein Member 2 *Australopithecus* skeleton. *South African J Sci*. 2002; 98: 523–526.
109. Partridge TC, et al. Lower Pliocene hominid remains from Sterkfontein. *Science*. 2003; 300: 607–12.
110. Harcourt-Smith W, Aiello L. Fossils, feet and the evolution of human bipedal locomotion. *J Anat*. 2004; 204: 403–416.
111. Arambourg C, Coppens Y. Découverte d'un australopithécien nouveau dans les gisements de l'Omo (Éthiopie). *South African J Sci*. 1968; 64: 58–59.
112. Chamberlain AT, Wood BA. A reappraisal of the variation in hominid mandibular corpus dimensions. *Am J Phys Anthrop*. 1985; 66: 399–403.
113. Asfaw B, et al. *Australopithecus garhi:* A new species of early hominid from Ethiopia. *Science*. 1999; 284: 629–635.
114. Leakey LSB. A new fossil skull from Olduvai. *Nature*. 1959; 184: 491–493.
115. Robinson JT. The affinities of the new Olduvai australopithecine. *Nature*. 1960; 186: 456–458.

116. Wood BA, Wood C, Konigsberg L. *Paranthropus boisei*: An example of evolutionary stasis? *Am J Phys Anthrop*. 1994; 95: 117–136.

117. Broom R. The Pleistocene anthropoid apes of South Africa. *Nature*. 1938; 142: 377–379.

118. Volkov T. Variations squelettiques du pied chez les primates et dans les races humaines. *Bull Soc Anthrop Paris*. 1903; 632–708.

119. Duckworth WLH. Description of a foetus of *Gorilla savagei*. In: *Studies from the Anthropological Laboratory*. Cambridge: Anatomy School; 1904: 41–50.

120. Volkov T. Variations squelettiques du pied chez les primates et dans les races humaines. *Bull Soc Anthrop Paris*. 1904; 1–50, 201–331, 720–725.

121. Straus WL. The growth of the human foot and its evolutionary significance. *Contrib Embryol*. 1927; 101: 93–134.

122. Lisowski F. Growth changes and comparisons of the primate talus with a note of clinical findings. *Ethiopian Med J*. 1966; 4: 173–179.

123. Lisowski FP. Angular growth changes and comparisons in the primate talus. *Folia Primatol*. 1967; 7: 81–97.

124. Day MH, Wood BA. Functional affininities of the Olduvai hominid 8 talus. *Man*. 1968; 3: 440–455.

125. Clarke RJ, Tobias PV. Sterkfontein Member 2 foot bones of the oldest South African hominid. *Science*. 1995; 269: 521–524.

126. Kidd KS, O'Higgins P, Oxnard CE. The OH8 foot: A reappraisal of the functional morphology of the hindfoot utilizing a multivariate analysis. *J Human Evol*. 1996; 31: 269–291.

127. Lewis OJ. The joints of the evolving foot. Part I. The ankle joint. *J Anat*. 1980; 130: 527–543.

128. Robinson J. *Early Hominid Posture and Locomotion*. Chicago: University of Chicago Press; 1972.

129. Le Gros Clark W. Observations on the anatomy of the fossil Australopithecinae. *J Anat*. 1947; 81: 300.

130. Susman RL. New hominid fossils from the Swartkrans Formation (1979–1986 excavations): Postcranial specimens. *Am J Phys Anthrop*. 1989; 79: 451–474.

131. Susman RL. Hominid postcranial remains from Swartkrans. In: Brain CK, ed. *Swartkrans: A Cave's Chronicles of Early Man*. Pretoria: Transvaal Museum; 1993: 117–136.

132. Susman R, Brain T. New first metatarsal (SKX 5017) from Swartkrans and the gait of *Paranthropus robustus. Am J Phys Anthrop*. 1988. 77: 7–15.

133. Tattersall I, Schwartz J. *Extinct Humans*. Boulder, CO: Westview; 2000: 89.

134. Campbell BG, Loy JD. *Humankind Emerging*. 7th ed. Boston: Allyn & Bacon, Pearson Education; 1996.

135. Susman RL, de Ruiter DJ. New hominin first metatarsal (SK 1813) from Swartkrans. *J Hum Evol*. 2004; 47: 171–181.

136. Day MH, Thornton CMB. The extremity bones of *Paranthropus robustus* from Kromdraai B, east Formation member 3, Republic of South Africa – A reappraisal. In: Mizerová A, ed. *Fossil Man. New Facts, New Ideas. Papers in Honor of Jan Jelínek's Life Anniversary*. Vol. 23. Brno: Anthropos; 1986: 91–99.

137. Broom R, Schepers GWH. The South African fossil ape-men, the *Australopithecinae. Transv Mus Mem*. 1946; 2:1–272.

138. Musgrave JH. *An Anatomical Study of the Hands of Pleistocene and Recent Man*. London: Cambridge University; 1970,

139. Day MH. Functional interpretations of the morphology of postcranial remains of early African hominids. In: Jolly C, ed. *Early Hominids of Africa*. London: Duckworth; 1978: 311–345.

140. Napier JR. The evolution of bipedal walking in the hominids. *Arch. Biol. (Liege)*. 1964; 75: 673–708.

141. Wood B, Collard M. The human genus. *Science*. 1999; 284: 65–71.

142. Leakey L, Tobias P, Napier J. A new species of the genus *Homo* from Olduvai Gorge. *Nature*, 1964; 202: 7.
143. Lewis OJ. Functional morphology of the joints of the evolving foot. *Symp Zool Soc London*. 1981; 46: 169–188.
144. Lisowski F, Albrecht G, Oxnard C. The form of the talus in some higher primates: A multivariate study. *Am J Phys Anthrop*. 1974; 41: 191–215.
145. Lisowski F, Albrecht G, Oxnard C. African foot tali: Further multivariate morphometric studies. *Am J Phys Anthrop*. 1976; 45: 5–18.
146. Susman R, Stern J. Functional morphology of *Homo habilis. Science*. 1982; 217: 931–933.
147. Bojsen-Møller F. Calcaneocuboid joint and stability of the longitudinal arch of the foot at high and low gear push off. *J Anat*. 1979; 129: 165–176.
148. Kidd R, O'Higgins P, Oxnard C. The OH 8 foot: A reappraisal of the functional morphology of the hindfoot utlizing a multivariate analysis. *J Human Evol*. 1996; 31: 269–291.
149. Kidd RS. On the nature of morphology: Selected canonical variates analyses of the hominoid hindtarsus and their interpretation. In: Jablonski NG, ed. *Shaping Primate Evolution*. Cambridge: Cambridge University Press; 2004.
150. Lewis O. Functional morphology of the joints of the evolving foot. *Symp Zool Soc London*. 1981a; 46: 169–188.
151. Oxnard C, Lisowski F. Functional articulation of some hominid foot bones: implications for the Olduvai (hominid 8) foot. *Am J Phys Anthrop*. 1980; 52: 107–117.
152. Harcourt-Smith WEH, Aiello L. An investigation into the degree of hallux abduction of the OH8 foot. *Am J Phys Anthrop Supplement*. 1999; 28: 145.
153. Day M, Napier J. Fossil foot bones. *Nature*. 1964; 201: 969.
154. Archibald J, Lovejoy C, Heiple K. Implications of relative robusticity in Olduvai metatarsus. *Am J Phys Anthrop*. 1972; 37: 93–96.
155. Day MH, Napier JR. A hominid toe bone from Bed I, Olduvai Gorge, Tanzania. *Nature*. 1966; 211: 929–930.
156. Day MH. Olduvai Hominid 10: A multivariate analysis. *Nature*. 1967; 215: 323–324.
157. Oxnard C. Some African fossil foot bones: A note on the interpolation of fossils into a matrix of extant species. *Am J Phys Anthrop*. 1972; 37: 3–12.
158. Lewis O. The joints of the evolving foot. Part III. The fossil evidence. *J. Anat*. 1980; 131: 275–298.
159. Susman RL, Stern JT. Functional morphology of *Homo habilis. Science*. 1982; 217: 931–934.
160. Henderson A, Wood B. The functional anatomy of the Olduvai (O.H. 8) foot [Abstract]. *J Anat Lond*. 1977; 124: 252.
161. Oxnard CE, Lisowski FP. Functional articulation of some hominoid foot bones: implications for the Olduvai (Hominid 8) foot. *Am J Phys Anthrop*. 1980; 52: 107–117.
162. Groves CP, Mazák V. An approach to the taxonomy of the Hominidae: Gracile Villafranchian hominids of Africa. *Cas Miner Geol*. 1975; 20: 225–247.
163. Day MH, Leakey REF. New evidence for the genus *Homo* from East Rudolf, Kenya. (III). *Am J Phys Anthrop*.1973; 41: 367–380.
164. Walker AC, Leakey, REF, eds. *The Nariokotome* Homo erectus *Skeleton*. Cambridge, MA: Harvard University Press; 1993: 457.
165. Gabunia L, Vekua A, Lordkipanidze D. The environmental contexts of early human occupation of Georgia (Transcaucasia). *J Human Evol*. 2000; 38: 785–802.
166. Gabunia L, de Lumley M-A, Berillon G. Morphologie et fonction due troisème métatarsien de Dmanisi, Géorgie orientale. In: Otte D, ed. *Early Humans at the Gates of Europe*. Liège: L' études et recherches archéologiques de l'Université de Liège; 2000: 29–41.
167. Antón SC. Natural history of *Homo erectus. Yrbk Phys Anthrop*. 2004; 46: 126–170.

168. Leonard WR, Robertson ML. Ecological correlates of home range variation in primates: implications for hominid evolution. In: Garber PA, ed. *On the Move: How and Why Animals Travel in Groups*. Chicago: University of Chicago Press; 2000: 628–648.

169. Ruff CB, Walker A. Body size and body shape. In: Leakey R, ed.*The Nariokotome Homo erectus Skeleton*. Cambridge: Harvard University Press; 1993: 234–265.

170. Gruss LT, Schmitt D. Bipedalism in *Homo ergaster*: An experimental study of the effects of tibial proportions on locomotor biomechanics. In: Hilton CE, ed. *From Biped to Strider: The Emergence of Modern Human Walking, Running, and Transport*. New York: Kluwer Academic/Plenum; 2004: 117–133.

171. Alexeev V. *The Origin of the Human Race*. Moscow: Progress; 1986.

172. Wood BA. Early hominid species and speciation. *J Human Evol*. 1992; 22: 351–365.

173. Dubois E. Palaeontologische andrezoekingen op Java. *Versl Mijnw Batavia*. 1892; 3: 10–14.

174. Weidenreich F. Some problems dealing with ancient man. *Am Anthrop*. 1940; 42: 375–383.

175. Bermúdez de Castro JM, et al. A hominid from the Lower Pleistocene of Atapuerca, Spain: Possible ancestor to Neandertals and modern humans. *Science*. 1997; 276: 1392–1395.

176. Lorenzo C, Arsuaga J-L, Carretero J-M. Hand and foot remains from the Gran Dolina Early Pleistocene site (Sierra de Atapuerca, Spain). *J Human Evol*.1999; 37: 501–522.

177. Schoetensack O. *Der Unterkierfer des Homo heidelbergensis aus den Sanden von Mauer bei Heidelberg*. Leipzig: W. Engelmann; 1908: 1–6.

178. Lamy P. *L'Homo Erectus et La Place De L'homme De Tautavel Parmi Les Hominidés Fossiles*. Paris: Congrès International de Paléontologie Humaine; 1982.

179. King W. The reputed fossil man of the Neanderthal. *Quart J Sci*.1864; 1: 88–97.

180. Krings M, et al. Neandertal DNA sequences and the origin of modern humans. *Cell*. 1997; 90: 19–30.

181. Krings M, et al. DNA sequence of the mitochondrial hypervariable region II from the Neandertal type specimen. *Proc Nat Acad Sci USA*. 1999; 96: 5581–5585.

182. Ovchinnikov IV, et al. Molecular analysis of Neanderthal DNA from the northern Caucasus. *Nature*. 2000; 404: 490–493.

183. Krings M, et al. A view of Neandertal genetic diversity. *Nature Genetics*. 2000; 26: 144–146.

184. Schmitz RW, et al. The Neandertal type site revisited: Interdisciplinary investigations of skeletal remains from the Neander Valley, Germany. *Proc Nat Acad Sci*. 2002; 99:13342–13347.

185. Serre D, et al. No evidence of Neandertal mtDNA contribution to early modern humans. *PloS*. 2004; 2: e57.

186. Rhoads JG, Trinkaus E. Morphometrics of the Neandertal talus. *Am J Phys Anthrop*. 1977; 46: 29–43.

187. Lisowski FP, Albrecht, GH, Oxnard CE. The form of the talus in some higher primates: A multivariate study. *Am J Phys Anthrop*.1974; 41: 191–216.

188. Trinkaus E. Squatting among the Neandertals: A problem in the behavioral interpretation of skeletal morphology. *J Archaeol Sci*.1975; 2: 327–351.

189. Trinkaus E. Functional aspects of Neandertal pedal remains. *Foot and Ankle*. 1983; 3: 377–390.

190. Trinkaus E. *A Functional Analysis of the Neandertal Foot*. University of Pennsylvania; 1975.

191. Boule M. L'homme fossil de La Chapelle-aux-Saints. *Ann. Paléont*. 1911; 6: 111–172.

192. Boule M. L'homme fossil de la Chapelle-aux-Saints. *Ann. Paléont*. 1912; 7: 3–192.

193. Boule M. L'homme fossil de la Chapelle-aux-Saints. *Ann. Paléont*. 1913; 8:1–67.

194. Morton DJ. Significant characteristics of the Neanderthal foot. *Nat. Hist*. 1926; 26: 310–314.

195. Trinkaus E, Hilton CE. Neandertal pedal proximal phalanges: Diaphyseal loading patterns. *J Human Evol*. 1996; 30: 399–425.

196. Tillier A-M. The evolution of modern humans: Evidence from young Mousterian individuals. In: Stringer CB, ed. *The Human Revolution*. Princeton, NJ: Edinburgh University Press; 1989: 286–297.

197. Rak Y, Kimbel WH, Hovers E. On Neandertal autapomorphies discernible in Neandertal infants: A response to Creed-Miles et al. *J Human Evol*.1996; 30: 155–158.
198. Brown P, et al. A new small-bodied hominin from the Late Pleistocene of Flores, Indonesia. *Nature*. 2004; 431: 1055–1061.
199. Linnaeus C. *Systema Naturae*. Stockholm: Laurentii Salvii; 1758.
200. White T, et al. Pleistocene *Homo sapiens* from Middle Awash, Ethiopia. *Nature*. 2003. 423: 742–747.
201. McDougall, I, Brown FH, Fleagle JG, Stratigraphic placement and age of modern humans from Kibish, Ethiopia. *Nature*. 2005; 433: 733–736.
202. Dreyer TF. A human skull from Florisbad, Orange Free State, with a note on the Endocranial Cast (by C. U. Ariëns-Kappers). *Proc Acad Sci Amst*. 1935; 38: 119–128.
203. Day MH, Stringer CB. Les restes crâniens d'Omo-Kibish et leur classification à l'intérieur du genre *Homo*. *L'Anthropologie*. 1991; 95: 73–594.
204. Pearson OM. Postcranial remains and the origins of modern humans. *Evol Anthrop*. 2000; 9: 229–247.
205. Rightmire GP, Deacon HJ. Comparative studies of late Pleistocene human remains from Klasies River Mouth, South Africa. *J Human Evol*. 1991; 20: 131–156.
206. Gebo DL. Schwartz GT. Foot bones from the Omo-implications for hominid evolution. *Am J Phys Anthrop*. in press.
207. Deloison Y. Description d'un calcanéum fossile de Primate et sa comparaison avec des calcanéums de Pongidés d'Australopitheques et d'*Homo*. *CR Acad Sci Paris*. 1986; 302 series III 685–692.
208. Deloison, Y. Description d'un astragale fossile de primate et comparaison avec des astragales de chimpanzés, de d'*Homo sapeins* et d'hominidés fossiles: Australopithéques et *Homo habilis*. *C.R. Acad Sci Paris*. 1997; 324 Series IIa: 685–692.

3
How the Foot Works

This chapter is a review of how we have reached our present state of knowledge of the human foot. The gross structure of the foot was known long before there was an understanding of how it functioned. These insights only started in the nineteenth century. They continue to be pursued thanks to the growth of biomechanical studies by orthopaedic surgeons and sports scientists.

Structure

Leonardo da Vinci (1452–1519) was especially interested in the manner in which individual muscles move the bones to which they are attached, but it is only fairly recently that English translations of his notebooks have become accessible. His drawings of the skeleton are among the outstanding features of his work [1]. He noted that the sesamoid bones were found near the insertions of tendons. It was thought by Rabbi Ushaia in 210 A.D. that the medial sesamoid, the larger of the two sesamoids that are embedded in the plantar plate beneath the head of the first metatarsal and provide a tunnel for the tendon of flexor hallucis longus, a bone of 'luz' or 'lus', was the nucleus from which resurrection would occur. The name 'sesamum' is said to have first been used by Galen about 180 A.D because these ossicles resembled the seeds of the plant *Sesamum indicum*, the oil of which was used as a purgative in ancient Rome [2]. The mechanical effect of the sesamoids of the great toe is shown in Figure 3.1. The task of writing an anatomical textbook based on observation was achieved by Andreas Vesalius of Brussels (1514–1564) [3]. The gross anatomy of the skeleton of the human foot was clearly set out by Vesalius when he published his book, *De humani corporis fabrica* (*On the Fabric of the Human Body*), in 1543 [4]. Illustrations based on his drawings were made from woodcuts by artists from the school of Titian 9 (see Figure 3.2). There were also the articulated bones of the foot as seen from above and below and various views of the talus, calcaneum, and navicular.

The terminology of the fingers was applied to the toes so that there is an index and ring toe, a classification that would be approved even today by medicolegal authorities. Muscles acting on the foot that are mentioned include tibiales anterior and posterior, and peronei longus and brevis. Vesalius noted that it is by means of the joint between the tibia, fibula, and talus that we flex and extend the foot. He describes how the round head of the talus encrusted with slippery cartilage articulated with a deep socket in the navicular. In his opinion it is at this joint

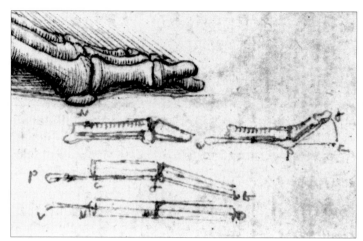

Figure 3.1. From drawing by Leonardo da Vinci to show the sesamoids of the great toe. (Reprinted by kind permission from the Royal Collection ©2004, Her Majesty Queen Elizabeth II.)

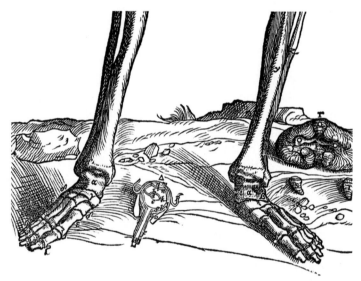

Figure 3.2. The feet as shown in *De humani corporis fabrica*, 1543 by Andreas Vesalius. (Reprinted by kind permission of the Wellcome Library, London.)

that the foot can perform a slight movement to either side. He mentioned that the toes like the fingers have three bones each, except the big toe which has only two. He suggested that this is so that the front of the hollow of the foot may rest more firmly on the ground [4]. The great toe was called the 'hallux,' the large toe, derived from the Greek, 'I spring or leap' [5].

Function

The next treatise on the function of the foot was presented in 1836 by the Weber brothers. One of them, Eduard Friederich (1806–1871), was an anatomist, and the other Wilhelm Eduard (1804–1891), was a mathematician and Professor of Physics at Gottingen. They produced the first comprehensive theory of walking and running in *Mechanik der menschlichen gehwerkzeuge* (*Mechanics of the Human Walking Apparatus*). With regard to the structure of the foot and mobility of its parts, they noted that the foot changes its shape so that it adapts to the contour of the ground when walking, so it always contacts the ground in several places. Secondly, the firmer part of the foot is used to lengthen the supporting leg when we stand on the bulk of the foot and as a result of the elastic binding of its components, potentially can dampen harmful shocks and make them harmless to the foot itself and the remainder of the body. They suggested that the function of the foot could be understood by using the analogy of a wheel.

> The foot by itself works as a small segment of a wheel, whereas the lower leg and the thigh behave together like spokes as in a wheel rolling on the ground, successive points on the wheel always come into contact with successive points on the ground, so that the wheel progresses without need of displacement or rubbing. The same process occurs for the plantar sole during walking. Rolling of the plantar sole thus consists of a successive shifting of pushing against the ground from the heel to the tip of the toes. As in a wheel, rolling avoids friction which would occur in displacement by sliding. Besides this advantage, rolling of the plantar sole on the ground during walking also provides the advantage that it considerably increases the step. . . . This rolling thus increases the step by the length of a foot. The forward foot strikes the ground with its heel and finally leaves the ground from its toes, after having rolled on the ground its whole length. Rolling of the plantar sole is a way of making steps longer and consequently, of using fewer steps in a given time for a consistent velocity of gait. This contributes to the comfort of walking. We would lack this advantage if our legs were built like stilts, which when striking and leaving the ground always rest with their tip at the same point and are provided with no surface for rolling.
>
> Weber and Weber [6]

James Gray in his classic book *How Animals Move* (1953) uses a similar analogy [7] (see Figure 3.3)

Henry Gray in the first edition of his book *Anatomy, Descriptive and Surgical* [8] in 1858 (it has now reached number thirty-eight), stated,

> The movements of the ankle are limited to flexion and extension. There is no lateral motion. The movements permitted between the bones of the first row, astragalus and os calcis are limited to a gliding upon each other, from before backwards, and from side to side. The gliding movement which takes place between the bones of the sec-

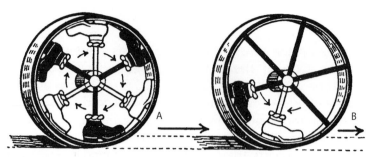

Figure 3.3. The foot as part of a wheel. (From James Gray How Animals Move (1953) Cambridge University Press, page 19, with permission)

ond row is very slight, the articulation between the scaphoid and cuneiform bones being more moveable than those of the cuneiforms with each other and with the cuboid. The movements which take place between the two rows is more extensive, and consists in a sort of rotation, by means of which the sole of the foot may be slightly flexed, and extended or carried inwards or outwards.

With regard to movement of the foot upon the leg, Humphry [9] wrote,

> . . . rarely do we contemplate anything more calculated to excite our admiration. Consider their variety, the rapidity with which they take place, in order to effect the requisite positions in walking and running, and to adapt the sole to the inequalities of the surface on which we tread; and remember the great weight has to be sustained while these movements are going on: yet how seldom is there a failure. . . .
>
> The movements that take place in the three joints of the foot are not so simple but very difficult to analyse and make out correctly. The difficulty is due, partly, to the close proximity of the joints to one another, which renders it no easy matter to distinguish the movements of one from another, and partly to the fact that the movements in each joint are a little oblique. . . . In the Human Skeleton, all the bones are bent and twisted, some in two or three directions; and the surfaces by which any bone is jointed to adjacent bones are invariably oblique with regard to each other.

However, in 1886, in a lecture recorded in *The Lancet* [10], Humphry stated,

> The astragaloscaphoid joint being a ball-and-socket joint would permit movement in any direction, but the movements are limited and determined by the ligaments and by the form of the articular surfaces of the calcaneocuboid joint with which it is associated, the two forming practically one joint resembling a hinge-joint; and the movements are thus reduced to flexion and extension, which take place on an oblique axis passing from within downwards and outwards through the middle of the ball of the astragalus and the forepart of the os calcis.

This must be one of the earliest descriptions of the axis of the midtarsal joint in English.

In order to estimate the angular displacement at a joint in any direction, it is customary to first determine the axis about which the movement is occurring [11]. Because at a typical joint this axis is not stationary, the concept of the fixed 'axis of a joint' is unsatisfactory, for during movement its position changes from one moment to the next. Nevertheless, it is usually possible to arrive at a 'compromise axis' that is the mean of all the momentary axes. The position of the compromise axis is sometimes unexpected. The axis at the subtalar joint might be thought to be directed in the long axis of the foot; in fact it is directed upwards and medially as well as forward as an inheritance from our primate relatives who walked with the soles of their feet facing inward gripping the branches of trees (in the supinated position). Once one knows the position of the axis, the movements and the arrangements of the muscles in this region are easy to understand.

The momentary axes at a joint are difficult to locate in life but they can be worked out post-mortem and the results transferred to the living subject. An accurate method was devised by Manter [12] (see Figure 3.4). Metal indicator pins are driven into the fixed and moving bones and the paths traced by their outer ends are used to deduce the momentary axes. This is a useful technique for investigating the movements at small joints such as those within the tarsus and has been successfully used by Verne T. Inman and his team [13] and Hicks [15]. The position of the axis of the ankle joint can be estimated by palpation of the tips of

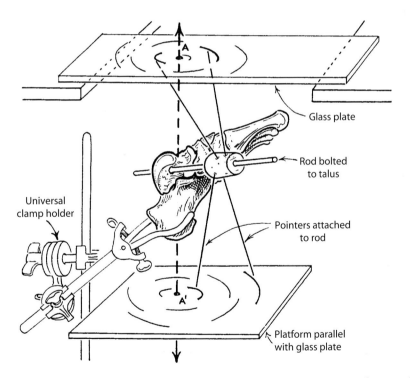

Figure 3.4. Apparatus used for determination of the axes of joints. Concentric arcs are traced on two platforms as the talus is turned at the subtalar joint. AA indicates the position of the axis of the joint. (From Manter JT. Movements of subtalar and transvers tarsal joints, The Anatomical Record 1941;80:397–410. Reprinted by permission of Wiley Liss, Inc., a subsidiary of John Wiley & Sons, Inc.)

the malleoli. It has been shown by Inman that it deviates slightly downwards and posteriorly when traced from medial to lateral. Inman stressed that it is the relationship between the ankle axis in the transverse plane and the midline of the foot that is functionally important. Inversion accompanies plantarflexion, and eversion is correlated with dorsiflexion. The adjoining surfaces of the fibula and talus tend to lose their correct degree of alignment as the foot is dorsiflexed. This explains the retention in man of mobile tibiofibular joints. In some animals the tibia and fibula are fixed and the lateral surface of the talus remains more or less perpendicular to the axis of the ankle joint whatever the position of the foot.

There is some controversy with regard to the axis of the ankle joint, particularly the clinical significance of a shift in direction close to the neutral position between plantarflexion and dorsiflexion observed by, among others, Barnett and Napier [14] (Figure 3.5A, B) and Hicks [15]. The axis of the ankle joint is not fixed and horizontal, but is inclined downwards and laterally during dorsiflexion, and downwards and medially during plantarflexion. The change occurs within a few degrees of the neutral position of the talus.

In 1989 movements of the ankle were measured using roentgen stereophotogrammetry in eight healthy volunteers with 0.8 mm tantalum marker beads [16]. These were 'shot' into the tibia, talus, calcaneum, medial cuneiform, and first metatarsal bones, so that they could be clearly seen in the region of the ankle

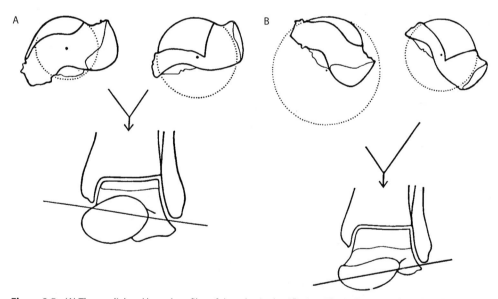

Figure 3.5. (A) The medial and lateral profiles of the talus in dorsiflexion. The inclination of the dorsiflexion axis downwards and laterally is obtained by joining the axes of rotation. (B) The medial and lateral profiles of the talus in plantarflexion. The inclination of the plantar axis (downwards and medially) is obtained by joining the centres of rotation. (Reprinted from Barnett C, Napier JR. The axis of rotation of the ankle joint in man. Journal of Anatomy 1952;86:1–9, with permission from Blackwell Publishing.)

joint. The results showed that the axis of the ankle changes continuously throughout weight-bearing movement. In dorsiflexion, as shown by Barnett and Napier in 1952 [14], it tended to be oblique downward and laterally. With rotation of the leg, the axis was variously inclined between the horizontal and the vertical. All axes in each subject lay close to the midpoint of a line between the tips of the malleoli. This study showed that the axis of the ankle joint may alter considerably during the arc of movement and differ significantly between individuals. When the axes of plantarflexion, dorsiflexion, pronation, supination, and medial and lateral rotation for each subject were drawn in the same figure, all axes irrespective of their inclination coincide or run very close to one central point in the trochlea of the talus (Figure 3.6). This may indicate the existence of a centre of rotation in the ankle joint.

The Subtalar Joint

As pointed out by Inman, the talus plays a unique role in the functional anatomy of the lower extremity. It is the link between the leg and the foot. The ankle joint is its proximal connection to the leg and the subtalar joint (sometimes called lower ankle joint) is its distal connection to the foot. In addition, movement of the talus produces important and definitive effects upon the foot through its distal articulation with the navicular.

Inman surveyed the European literature in detail. He gives credit to Meyer (1853) [17] writing in German for providing the first clear description of the axis of rotation, including its position as projected in the sagittal and transverse

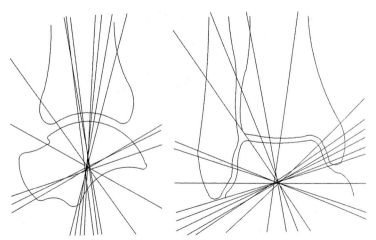

Figure 3.6. All coronal and sagittal plane projections of plantarflexion and dorsiflexion, pronation and supination, and medial and lateral rotation axes tend to meet in one small area of the talus. (Reprinted with permission from Lundberg A, Svensson OK, Nemeth G, et al. The axis of rotation of the ankle joint. J Bone Joint Surg Br. 1989 Jan;71(1):94–9.)

planes. The axis of the subtalar joint was also described in *Quain's Elements of Anatomy* in 1892 [18]. Elftman and Manter in 1935 [19] expanded the concept that movement between talus and calcaneum was about an oblique axis. Manter (1941) reported the average inclination of the subtalar axis to be 42 degrees projected onto the sagittal plane and deviating anteriorly and medially by 16 degrees in the horizontal plane. This work was supported by Inman who agreed with their findings but found more individual variation.

Manter [12] was most specific that the movement of the talus on the calcaneum is accompanied by a longitudinal displacement and therefore the movement resembles that of a screw. The plane of rotation of the subtalar joint was found, upon measurement, to lie on a slant with respect to the axis. Consequently, the movement of the joint consists of rotation in a direction oblique to the axis of the joint. Because sideways slipping does not occur, the action of the subtalar joint is very like that of a screw. The subtalar joint behaves like a right-handed screw in the right foot and a left-handed one in the left foot. Inman considered it reasonable to assume that in approximately one half of the population, movement at the subtalar joint results in some linear displacement of the talus along the joint axis but the pitch of the screwing movement varies widely from individual to individual. In the other half of the population the movement is not like a screw and the talus may or may not be displaced forward or backward when there is movement between the talus and calcaneum.

The action of the talocalcaneal (subtalar) joint is likened by Inman to a mitred hinge connecting the leg to the foot. Within a limited range longitudinal rotation of the leg imposes a longitudinal rotation of the foot (supination and pronation) which is passive at heel strike, and active at toe off; it is also a directional torque converter.

The subtalar axis as described and illustrated is a 'compromise axis' [19]. This axis could only be fixed and stationary if the component rotations of the inversion–eversion movement in three body planes took place simultaneously and in a constant ratio. For most joints it is improbable that this would be the case. Van Langelaan [21] has shown a fairly closely aggregated bundle or sheaf of momentary axes is necessary to depict the movement accurately throughout its different phases (see Figure 3.7). Although a single axis may not define the movement with mechanical precision, it nevertheless represents the pattern of the movement as a whole. The obliquity of this axis gives the subtalar joint its most significant properties. Indispensable for our ancestors in tree climbing it allows us to adjust our feet on rough ground. Its large component of vertical rotation gives the possibility of transverse rotation at the ankle under the control of gravity [22].

The Midtarsal or Transverse Tarsal Joint

This lies immediately in front of the talus and calcaneum and is connected to the hindfoot by the talonavicular and calcaneocuboid joints. Although the cuboid and

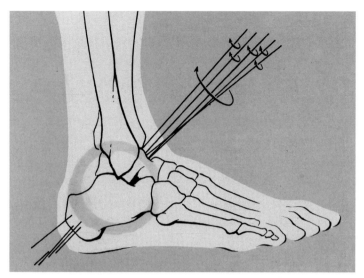

Figure 3.7. A sheaf of axes as suggested by Van Langelaan. (Reprinted with permission from [21].)

navicular bones are not rigidly attached to each other, any relative movement between them is so minor that we are entitled to consider the two bones as moving together. It is at this joint that changes in the height of the longitudinal arch occur. Elftman [23] demonstrated that the axes of these two joints are parallel when the calcaneum is everted so that the foot is as flexible as possible to be an effective shock absorber during the loading response at midstance in the gait cycle. When the axes are not parallel there is rigidity at the midtarsal joint at toe-off when the foot is supinated so that it can act as an effective lever for propulsion (see Figure 3.8).

How the Longitudinal Arch Works

Humphry [24] stated,

You may think that the arch of the foot would have been a much simpler structure, as well as stronger, if it had been composed of one bone instead of several. But it must be remembered that it would, then, have been liable to be cracked and broken by the sudden and violent manner in which during running and jumping, the weight of the body is thrown upon it.

Moreover, the several bones where they touch one another are covered with a tolerably thick layer of highly elastic gristle or cartilage; and this provision together with the slight movements which take place between these bones give an elasticity to the foot and to the step, and serves to break the jars and shocks caused by the sudden contact of the foot with the ground.

In *Quain's Anatomy* of 1892 [18] a transverse and longitudinal arch are mentioned, both capable by pressure from above of 'securing elasticity.' Professor

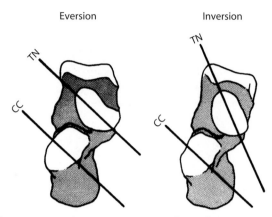

Eversion   Inversion

Figure 3.8. Function of transverse tarsal joint as described by Elftman, demonstrates that when the calcaneum is in eversion the resultant axes of the talonavicular (TN) and calcaneocuboid (CC) joints are parallel. When the subtalar joint is inverted the axes are not parallel and give increased stability to the midfoot. (Reprinted from Surgery of the Foot and Anke, 7 ed, Coughlin MJ, Mann RA, page 19, © 1999, with permission from Elsevier.)

McNeill Alexander, a zoologist interested in elastic mechanisms in animal movement, has shown experimentally as recently as 1987 using human amputated feet [25] loaded in a rig to simulate weight-bearing, that strain energy is stored in the foot and largely returned in an elastic recoil: the foot behaves like a spring. The graph of force against displacement shows a fairly narrow hysteresis loop (see Figure 3.9). He cut the ligaments supporting the arch in turn and found that the plantar aponeurosis, the long and short plantar ligaments, and the spring ligament are all important in the energy-storing mechanism either as stores of strain energy or by their roles in maintaining the integrity of the arch. He also noted that distortion of the hindfoot similar to flattening of the human arch has been demonstrated in running camels. There is no difference histologically between ligamentous structures of the foot and the plantar fascia [26]. They are composed of collagen and elastic fibres. The elastic fibres are numerous, show considerable difference in thickness, and are arranged predominantly in strands and bundlelike networks. Both the collagen and elastic fibres changed from a wavy to a straight configuration as stress was applied to specimens of plantar fascia [27].

The plantar fascia, which is morphologically the insertion of the plantaris muscle, has been shown by Hicks [28] to raise the longitudinal arch when the toes are dorsiflexed; the maximum effect is on the first ray and gradually diminishes laterally (the windlass mechanism). This is a passive mechanism with no muscular contraction. The stretched plantar fascia also inverts the calcaneum and rotates the tibia laterally. There is also the reverse effect when the arch is flattened under body weight so that the proximal phalanges become plantarflexed and the toes are firmly opposed to the ground. As pointed out by Stainsby [29] the transverse tie bar made up of the plantar plates and deep

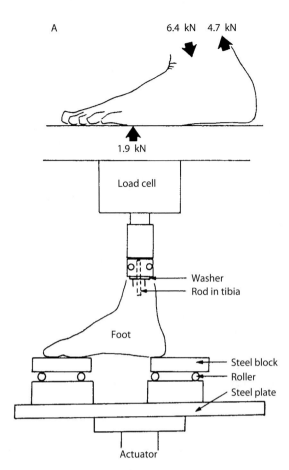

A

6.4 kN   4.7 kN

1.9 kN

Load cell

Washer
Rod in tibia

Foot

Steel block
Roller
Steel plate

Actuator

Figure 3.9. (A) Showing rig for loading a cadaveric foot; (B) showing hysteresis loop and relationship of strain energy to peak load. (Reprinted with permission from Ker RF, Bennett MB, Bibby SR et al. The spring in the arch of the human foot. Nature. 1987; 325 (7000):147–9.)

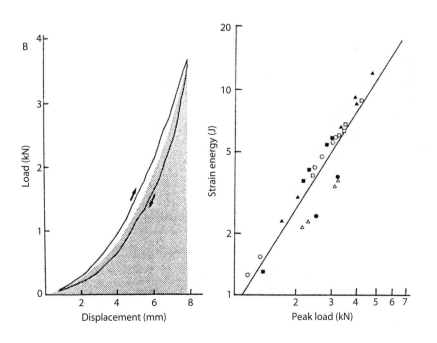

B

Load (kN)

Displacement (mm)

Strain energy (J)

Peak load (kN)

transverse metatarsal ligaments is connected to the plantar fascia and tightens on weight bearing to prevent splaying of the forefoot. Recently [30] the elastic properties of the plantar fascia during the contact phase of walking were determined experimentally by integrating a pressure-sensitive optical gait platform with a radiographic fluoroscopy system for recording movement of the bones of the foot. In order to calculate the ratio of tension in the fascia in relation to deformation, lateral images of the foot that allowed evaluation of the length of the fascia from arch-contact (i.e., full foot to toe-off) were obtained simultaneously with the vertical ground contact forces. In two women volunteers of similar physical proportions the plantar fascia was shown to undergo continuous elongation from arch-contact to toe-off, reaching a deformation of 9 to 12% between these positions. Rapid elongation of the plantar fascia was observed before and immediately after midstance, and a significantly slower elongation occurred around push-off and toe-off.

Flat Feet

The significance of the height of the longitudinal arch of the foot was a controversial issue in orthopaedic surgery for many years. A low arch or flat foot on weight bearing has traditionally been regarded as undesirable. Jones and Lovett in their textbook in 1923 [31] quote an investigation by Hoffman in 1907 [32] of 800 subjects of different racial origins. Hoffman concluded that there is no normal type of arch, that the height and shape of the arch are of no value in estimating the strength or usefulness of the foot, and that normal feet have high, medium, and low arches in the same proportion, as do feet with painful arches. The survey of 3619 soldiers in the Canadian Army by Harris and Beath in 1947 was a signal contribution to understanding flat feet [33]. They stated, 'It is evident that we cannot be content merely to recognise the deformity of flat foot. Our concern is with function. If this is good it matters little whether the longitudinal arch is depressed.'

Further, more recent work with measurements has clearly shown that flat feet are within the range of normal biological variability and should be considered physiologically normal [34,35]. Both these investigators used indices derived from measurements of the ratio of the width of the foot in the area of the arch and the width at the heel using Harris and Beath mats for footprints. Staheli et al. [35] showed that flat feet are usual in infants, common in children, and within the normal range of observations made in adult feet

Vibrations in the Human Skeleton

The impact of the foot with the ground sets the skeleton vibrating. Light et al. [36] used accelerometers to record these vibrations, at two points in the body of

McLellan, Volunteer and co-author. One accelerometer was attached to a bar which he held between his teeth to record vibrations in his skull. The other was attached to his tibia by a thin wire passed through the tibial tuberosity under local anaesthesia.

The predominant frequencies in the records are 20 to 50 Hz. The patterns of acceleration of tibia and teeth are similar, but the vibrations in the teeth occur about 10 ms later and only have about 20% of the amplitude of those of the tibia. The waves appear to be transmitted through the skeleton, losing amplitude as they travel.

All the records were made while walking on a hard laboratory floor. The largest accelerations occurred when McLellan walked barefoot or in shoes with hard leather heels. Both the amplitude and the frequency were reduced when he wore crepe-soled shoes, or shoes with a shock-absorbing insert in the heel. This is consistent with measurements of ground forces in running with and without shoes. The phenomenon seen in the illustrations (see Figures 3.10 and 3.11) seems to be the propagation of a wave of elastic strain (i.e., a sound wave) through the body [37].

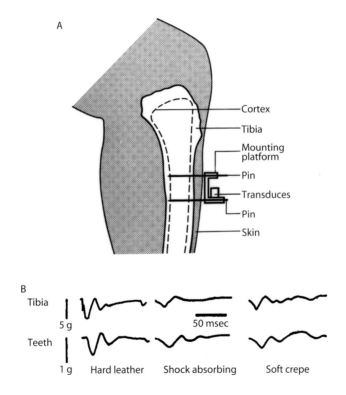

Figure 3.10. (A) To show transducer fixed to the tibia. (B) Waveform and order of magnitude of longitudinal acceleration transient on heel strike in normal walking. Simultaneous records from accelerometers attached to the tibia and held between the teeth when walking with three different soles. (Reprinted with permission from Light LH, McLellan GE, Klenerman L. Skeletal transients on heel strike in normal walking with different footwear. J Biomech. 1980;13(6):477–80.)

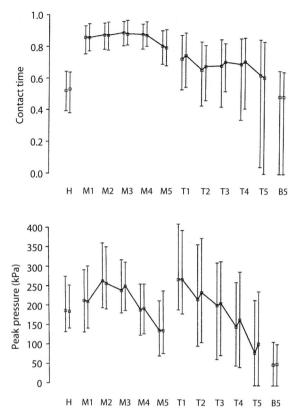

Figure 3.11. Contact time and peak pressures to show function of the toes. Above, the functions of the toes during the stance phase. The median (–) and 90% data interval (vertical bars) for contact time as a proportion of stance phase for left and right feet (left and right pairs of points) for all subjects for all areas examined; below for dynamic peak pressure for left and right feet (left and right pairs of points) for adults only for all areas examined (H: heel; M1–5: metatarsal heads; T1–5: great to fifth toe; B5: base of fifth metatarsal). (Reprinted with permission from Hughes J, Clark P, Klenerman L. The importance of the toes in walking. J Bone Joint Surg Br. 1990;72(2):245–51.)

Shock Absorption

The shock-absorbing capacity of the foot is thought to relate to its structure, particularly the height of the medial longitudinal arch. During running the ground reaction force may exceed several times body weight [38]. The foot sustains this force and reduces the likelihood of injury by deforming on striking the ground. In addition to the basic structural design of the foot there are other mechanisms which assist shock absorption. These are both active and passive. The passive mechanisms are the elasticity of bone and soft tissue, and the attenuating properties of articular cartilage and synovial fluid. Two important contributions to the absorption of energy are the fat pads at the heel and beneath the metatarsal heads. All activity of the joints of the foot is linked with proprioception and muscle activity [39]. An important example is the pre-activation of the stabilising muscles around the foot which control pronation. The height of the medial longitudinal arch is the main measurable structural characteristic of the foot and has been used in epidemiological studies of injury.

Giladi et al. [40] in a study of 295 military recruits noted a significant decrease in the number of stress fractures in subjects with a low arch as compared with a high arch. Further detail was provided by Simkin et al. [41] who demonstrated that compared with people with highly arched feet, subjects with low arches sustain a higher number of stress fractures in the metatarsals but they have a lower incidence of stress fractures in the long bones of the leg when compared to subjects with a high arch. This suggests that low-arched feet are more flexible and so more shock absorption occurs in the area of the foot than in high-arched feet as the latter are relatively more rigid and thus transfer the force more directly up the limb to the rest of the body. Despite clinical evidence relating the height of the medial longitudinal arch to injury it has not been possible to relate measured forces acting on the foot in walking or running to variations in arch height. A group of 18 normal athletic adult volunteers with clinically normal feet were investigated using a Kistler force platform. An Arch Index was calculated from lateral radiographs taken of the weight-bearing foot. Each subject performed ten trials running at a speed of 3 m using a forefoot running style.

The dynamic load rate showed three definite peaks and two intervening troughs showing that the process of shock absorption was one which was progressive and associated with several different mechanisms. However, none of the force peaks or load rate peaks correlated with the Arch Index [42].

The Importance of the Toes in Walking

In 1932 Lambrinudi [43] described the main functions of the toes as prehensile or ambulatory. Because modern humans rarely use their toes for gripping surfaces or objects, the main function of the toes is to improve leverage and enlarge the weight-bearing area so that at whatever height the heel is raised full body weight is not taken on the metatarsal heads alone. Lambrinudi stated that this mechanism was only effective if the toes were maintained flat on the ground with the intrinsic muscles contracting synergistically with the long flexors, and he predicted a reduction of function of the toes where deformities were present. His views were based on clinical observation and could not be substantiated by objective measurements.

Using a dynamic pedobarograph to which the Sheffield system of computerised analysis had been added, 160 normal subjects aged from five to seventy-eight years with no foot problems were investigated [44]. The toes were not in contact with the floor as long as the metatarsal heads but they were in contact with the substrate longer than the heel and the base of the fifth metatarsal. There was a decrease in median contact time between the great and fifth toes with a plateau in the middle. In 92% of subjects, contact was made with all the toes of both feet. The remaining 8% made no contact with the ground with one or more toes (usually the fifth).

The great toe reached the highest peak pressure recorded under the whole foot and the central toes took more pressure than the lateral metatarsal heads. The great toe took over half the force under the toes, followed by the second, third, fourth, and fifth toes. The area of the foot in contact with the ground can be seen to be less at toe-off than at heel strike. Thus although the force on the forefoot increases at the second peak of vertical loading, the area that takes the load decreases. Lambrinudi's observations have thus been confirmed by objective measurement. The toes are in contact with the ground for about three quarters of the walking cycle and exert pressure similar to that from the metatarsal heads (see Figures 3.11, 3.12 and 3.13).

The Sole

We do not see our soles which are out of sight and covered by thick skin, but yet they are of great importance for our posture and gait.

Recent work has reinforced the old adage, 'Keep your feet on the ground.' The plantar sole has been recognised as a 'dynamometric map' for control of human balance [45]. Numerous studies support the important contribution of sensation for the sole in the control of balance [46,47]. To stay upright we use exquisitely complicated and delicate feedback control, which works through the peripheral and central

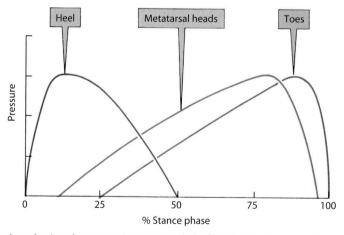

Figure 3.12. To show the time the toes are in contact with the floor during the stance phase.

nervous systems. It has also been stated that 'Besides their mechanical tasks, the feet at the ball and the heel, act as two antennae that repeatedly scan the ground' [48].

The concept of proprioception (perception of one's own) was introduced by Sir Charles Sherrington (1857–1952), Professor of Physiology at Liverpool and later at Oxford. He gave the name proprioreceptor to the receptor mechanisms which lie embedded within the deeper tissues, particularly muscles, tendons, and joints. These mechanisms can be distinguished from exteroreceptors, which lie near the surface of the body as, for example, the eye, ear, and skin. Sherrington and Ruffini in 1892 and 1893 demonstrated the sensory nature of 'muscle spindles' which are found in muscle. The demonstration of the sensory nature of the muscle spindle is fundamental to understanding the mechanism of the posture of the body and its relationship to tendons and muscle tone. It was proof that muscles and the deeper tissues are amply supplied with sense organs and from half to one third of a so-called motor nerve is made up of sensory fibres whose cell bodies are in the dorsal root ganglion [49].

There are four types of mechanoreceptors in the sole of the foot [50]. Merkel discs and Meissner's corpuscles are found in the superficial layers of the skin. Merkel discs are rapidly adapting receptors sensitive to vertical pressure (see Figure 3.13). Meissner's corpuscles are sensitive to local pressure, but adapt slowly allowing for maintenance of pressure sensitivity. Deep to the above are Ruffini and Pacinian receptors. Ruffini endings are sensitive to unidirectional skin stretch, whereas the Pacinian receptors are sensitive to rapid tissue movements. It is likely that impulses from the mechanoreceptors of the ankle also subserve a proprioceptive function [51].

As pointed out by Paul Brand [52], there are two types of nerve endings in the plantar skin that respond to mechanical force by a sense of pain but under very different conditions. One type is called a high threshold mechanorecep-tor. Impulses are carried by A-delta fibres and they give pain sensation in response to relatively high levels of force and pressure that impinge on healthy tissue. The other types are called polymodal nociceptors. These respond to mechanical stresses by generating severe pain at much lower thresholds of force, but only if they have already been activated by chemical production of inflammation or actual damage to living cells. The pressure of every step exceeds the low mechanical threshold of the polymodal nocicep-tors but we do not feel pain because they are not activated unless there is tis-sue damage. The pain from polymodal nociceptors forces one to limp or stop walking as soon as they are activated by the accumulated stresses and tissue damage that remain within the boundary of the permissive high-threshold mechanosystem. People with full sensation are protected from injury by the alternations of the two systems.

Brand concluded that three factors determine the probability of actual break-down and ulceration of the foot when there is loss of the sensation of pain. The

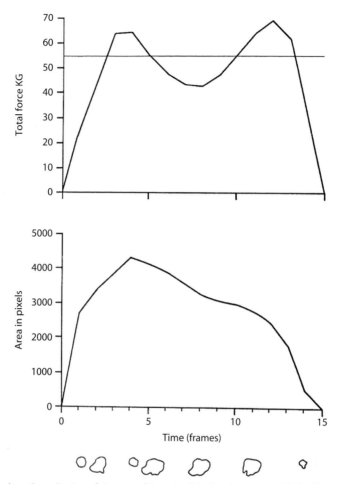

Figure 3.13. To show the reduction of the area of the sole of the foot in contact with the floor in relation to vertical pressure. Total force (above) and area of foot in contact with the ground (below) for a single foot plotted against time. (Reprinted with permission from Hughes J, Clark P, Klenerman L. The importance of the toes in walking. J Bone Joint Surg Br. 1990;72(2):245–51.)

first is the severity of the sensory loss and its localisation on the sole of the foot. The second is the magnitude of the forces that impinge on various parts of the sole of the foot while walking in normal footwear or in footwear that has been modified to spread the load and minimise the stress on areas of severe sensory loss. The third is the walking distance that it takes for moderate repetitive stress to build up a state of inflammation.

Somatosensory function declines with age and some changes have been associated with diminished motor performance and loss of balance. Vibrating gel-based insoles result in a reduction of all the variants of sway of the centre of gravity in elderly subjects. Thus it has been suggested that randomly vibrating insoles in shoes might be effective for the enhancement of dynamic activities of balance such as walking and could help elderly adults overcome postural instability caused by age-related sensory loss [53] and help in the reduction of falls and their consequences.

In a similar manner it has been found that wearing textured insoles in football boots improves the sensory feedback with regard to position of the foot [54]. The material used was a rubber sheeting with four nodules (3 mm high and 1 mm in diameter) per square centimetre. The relative sensory insulation provided by the modern running shoe has also been blamed for the frequency of injuries in athletes [55].

Summary

The details of how the foot works have gradually been accumulated over hundreds of years, at first by careful observation of the gross anatomy coupled with mathematical analysis. Later research was more quantitative and used more sophisticated biomechanical and radiological techniques. At the same time improved knowledge of the nervous system has helped our understanding of the dynamic function of the foot. More advanced imaging methods and computerised modelling are now available for further research on foot function.

References

1. O' Malley CD, Saunders JB. *Leonardo da Vinci on the Human Body*. New York: Henry Schuman; 1952: 27.
2. Helal B. The great toe sesamoid bones: The lus or lost souls of Ushaia. *Clin Orthopaed Related Res*. 1981; 157: 82–87.
3. Singer C, Underwood EA. *A Short History of Medicine*. London: Clarendon; 1962: 90.
4. Vesalius A. *On the Fabric of the Human Body. A Translation of De Humani Corporis Fabrica Libri Septem*. Richardson WF, Carman JB. San Francisco: Norman; 1998: 338–339.
5. Diab M. *Lexicon of Orthopaedic Etymology*. Amsterdam: Harwood Academic; 1999.
6. Weber W, Weber E. *Mechanics of the Human Walking Apparatus*. Translated from the German by Maquet P, Furlong R. Berlin: Springer Verlag; 1992: 17, 96.
7. Gray H. *How Animals Move*. Cambridge: Cambridge Press; 1953: 19.
8. Gray H. *Anatomy Descriptive and Surgical*. West Strand, London: Parker, John W, & Son; 1858: 178.
9. Humphry GM. *The Human Foot and the Human Hand*. Macmillan: Cambridge; 1861: 33,36.
10. Humphry, GM. Flat foot and the construction of the plantar arch. *The Lancet*. 1886; 529–531.
11. Barnett CH, Davies DV, Mac Conaill MA. *Synovial Joints*. London: Longmans Green; 1961: 253.
12. Manter JT, Movements of the subtalar and transverse tarsal joints. *Anat Rec*. 1941; 80: 397–410.
13. Inman VT. *The Joints of the Ankle*. Baltimore, MD: Williams and Wilkins; 1976.
14. Barnett CH, Napier JR. The axis of rotation of the ankle joint in man. *J Anat Lond*. 1952; 86: 1–9.
15. Hicks JH. The mechanics of the foot. *J Anat*. 1953; 87: 345–359.

16. Lundberg A, Svensson OK, Nemeth G, Selink G. The axis of rotation of the ankle joint. *J Bone Joint Surg (Br)*. 1989; 71B: 94–99.
17. Meyer H. Zweiter Beitrag zur Mechanick des menschlicken knochengerustes. *Arch Anat Physiol wissensch Med*. 1853; 365.
18. Schafer EA, Thane GD, eds. *Quains Elements of Anatomy*. Vol 2, part 2. 10th ed. London: Longman Green; 1892: 185.
19. Elftman H, Manter J. The evolution of the human foot with especial reference to the joints. *J Anat*. 1935; 70: 56–57.
20. Lewis OJ. *Functional Morphology of the Evolving Hand and Foot*. Oxford: Clarendon; 1989: 223.
21. Van Langelaan E J. A kinematical analysis of the tarsal joints. *Acta Orthopaed Scand*. 1983; 54(suppl 204): 11–269.
22. Elftman H. Dynamic structure of the human foot. *Artif Limbs*. 1969; 13: 49–58.
23. Elftman H. The transverse tarsal joint and its control. *Clin Orthopaed*. 1960; 16: 41–46.
24. Humphry GM. *The Human Foot and the Human Hand*. Cambridge: Macmillan; 1861: 18–19.
25. Ker RF, Dimery NJ, Alexander McNeill R. The spring in the arch of the human foot. *Nature*. 1987; 325, 147–149.
26. Wright DG, Rennels DC. A study of the elastic properties of plantar fascia. *J Bone Joint Surg*. 1964; 46A: 482–492.
27. Straub H. Die elastischen Fasern in den Bandern des menschlichen Fusses. *Acta Anat*.1950–1951; 11: 268–289.
28. Hicks JH. The mechanics of the foot II. The plantar aponeurosis and the arch. *J Anat*. 1954; 88: 25–30.
29. Stainsby GD. Pathological anatomy and dynamic effect of the displaced plantar plates and the importance of the plantar plate – Deep transverse metatarsal ligament tie bar. *Ann Roy Coll Surg*. 1997; 79: 58–68.
30. Gefen A. The in vivo elastic properties of the plantar fascia during the contact phase of walking. *Foot Ankle Int*. 2003; 24: 238–244
31. Jones R, Lovett RW. *Orthopaedic Surgery*. London: Henry Frowder and Hodder & Stoughton; 1923: 606.
32. Hoffmann P. Conclusions drawn from a comparative study of feet of barefooted and shoe wearing peoples. *Am J Orthopaed Surg*. 1905; iii: 105–135.
33. Harris RI, Beath T. *Army Foot Survey*. Vol. I. Ottawa: National Research Council of Canada; 1947.
34. Rose GK, Welton EA, Marshal T. The diagnosis of the flat foot in the child. *J Bone Joint Surg*. 1985; 67B: 426–428.
35. Staheli L, Chew D, Corbett M. The longitudinal arch. *J Bone Joint Surg*.1987; 69A: 71–78.
36. Light L, McLellan GE, Klenerman L. Skeletal transients of heel strike in normal walking with different footwear. *J Biomech*.1980; 13: 477–480.
37. Alexander McNeill R. *Elastic Mechanisms in Animal Movement*. Cambridge: Cambridge University Press; 1988: 105.
38. Cavanagh PR, La Fortune MA. Ground reaction forces in distance running. *J Biomech*. 1980; 13: 397–406.
39. Pratt DJ. Mechanism of shock alternation via the lower extremity during running. *Clin Biomech*. 1989; 4: 51–57.
40. Giladi M, Milgrom C, Stein M, Kashtan H, Margulies J, Chisin R, Stienberg R, Aharonson Z. The low arch, a protective factor in stress fractures. A prospective study in 295 military recruits. *Orthopaed Rev*. 1985; 14: 81–84.
41. Simkin A, Leichter L, Giladi M, Stein M, Milgrom C. Combined effect of foot arch structure and an orthotic device on stress fractures. *Foot and Ankle Int*. 1989; 10: 25–29.
42. Lees, A, Haynes A, Phillipson A, Klenerman, L. Shock absorption characteristics of the forefoot and its relationship to medial longitudinal arch height. *Foot Ankle Int* 2005; in press.

43. Lambrinudi C. Use and abuse of toes. *Postgrad. Med. J.* 1932; 8: 459–464.
44. Hughes J, Clarke P, Klenerman L. The importance of the toes in walking. *J Bone Joint Surg.* 1990; 72B: 245–251.
45. Kavoundiss A, Roll R, Roll J. The plantar sole in a "dynamometric map" for human balance control. *Neuro Rep.* 1998; 9: 3247–3252.
46. Watanabe I, Okubo J. The role of the plantar mechanoreceptor in equilibrium control. *Ann NY Acad Sci.* 1981; 374: 855–864.
47. Maki BE, Perry SD, Norrie RG, McEllroy W. Effect of facilitation of sensation from plantar foot–Surface boundaries on postural stabilis ation in young and older adults. *J Gerontol.* 1999; 54A: M281–287.
48. Bojsen-Moller, MF, Jorgensen L, Jahss, M. *Disorders of Foot and Ankle.* 2d ed. Philadelpia: WB Saunders Company; 1991: 532.
49. Fearing F. *Reflex Action, a Study in the History of Physiological Psychology.* Baltimore, MD: Williams and Wilkins; 1930: 219.
50. Riemin BL, Guskiewicz K, Lephart SM. Proprioception and neuromuscular control. In: Lephart MS, Fu FH, eds. *Joint Stability in Propriception and Neuromuscular Control in Joint Stability.* Champaign, IL: Human Kinetics; 2000: Chapter 4, 37.
51. Bertoff ES, Westerberg C. The mechanoreceptors of the sole of the foot and their clinical significance. *Acta Orthopaed. Scand.* 1988; 59: 101.
52. Brand PW. Tenderizing the foot. *Foot Ankle Int.* 2003; 24: 457–461.
53. Pripiata AA, Niemi JB, Harry JD, Lipeitz LA, Collins JJ. Vibrating insoles and balance control in elderly people. *The Lancet.* 2003; 362: 1123–1124.
54. Waddington G, Adams R. Football insoles and sensitivity to extent of ankle inversion movement. *Brit J Sports Med.* 2003; 37:170–175.
55. Robbins SE, Hanna AM. Running-related injury prevention through bare foot adaptations. *Med Sci Sports.* 1987; 19:148–156.
56. Coughlin MJ, Mann RA. *Surgery of the Foot and Ankle.* 7th ed. St Louis, MO: Mosby; 19.
57. Ker RF, Bennett MB, Bibby SR, et al. The spring in the arch of the human foot. *Nature.* 1987; 325 (7000): 147–149.

4
The Development of Gait

The patterns of activity of newborn mammals are appropriate to the environment into which they are born. In this respect mammals can be divided into four classes: herd animals, such as the horse, cow, and whale; nest animals, such as the lion, dog, and mouse; mother-clinging animals, such as primates, bats, and finally marsupials. Herd animals must be born in a state of relative 'maturity' to be able to follow the herd shortly after birth. When an animal is born into the security of a nest, there are advantages in birth at an early stage of development because a large bulk will be a handicap. A large baby needs more energy and this is difficult to obtain from diet alone. The young need only to feel their way to the mother's nipples for milk and for this purpose do not need a full complement of sensory apparatus nor full powers of locomotion.

Man, clearly a mother-clinging animal in an evolutionary context, has become a sort of nest animal [1]. The reasons for the usual 12-month interval between birth and independent walking and the additional two years required for maturation of gait, is probably a combination of the slower development of the motor system in humans and also the need for learning. The process of maturation, which leads to walking, is complex. Learning, emergence of cortical control, sensory integration, and myelination are taking place simultaneously. Cortical control and sensory integration occur because the necessary pathways become myelinated and functional.

The long postnatal period required for the development of walking cannot be due to lack of neuronal development. The brain of a full-term infant is already a quarter of the weight of the adult brain and is proportionately more mature at birth than other organs. Most neurons are present by seven and a half months from conception. The transformation of immature to mature walking follows an orderly pattern, which is best explained by progressive myelination. The timetable for myelination and the development of complex motor functions, including walking, are roughly parallel. Maturation of the motor system is the key factor in independent walking and the process of transformation of the shaky staccato movements of the toddler into the smooth energy-efficient pattern of mature walking [2]. The benefits of myelination include: lower energy requirements for nerve conduction, rapid conduction, and marked reduction in space required. Myelin, named and described by the German pathologist Rudolf Virchow in 1864, functions as an electrical insulator that speeds conduction with a relatively small nerve fibre, thus allowing a larger number of fibres in a small space. A much reduced flow of sodium ions is required with myelin present and the conduction signal leaps from one node of Ranvier to the next, saltatory conduction. Without myelin the entire axonal membrane must depolarise and then repolarise which is a much slower process [3].

Prenatal Movements

The development of real-time ultrasound techniques allows quantitative measurement of early foetal movement. The first movements occur 7 to 8.5 weeks after the last menstrual period They consist of 0.5 to 2 second periods of generalised shifting of the foetal contours. Subsequently the repertoire of movements increases rapidly. For example, at 15 weeks at least 15 distinct patterns can be recognised, such as isolated arm, leg, and head movements and hand–face contact.

The foetus starts to rotate around its sagittal or transverse axis after 11 weeks of gestation. A complete change in position can then be achieved by complex general movements, including alternating leg movements, which resemble infant stepping. These leg movements denote the first time during human ontogeny that movements like walking can be made [4].

The Infant

According to Peiper(1962) [5] the development of an erect gait takes place in different ingenious interlocking stages. The child is thus able to achieve tasks of increasing complexity. Progress is made by the strong urge for movement and activity which continually drives the child to new experiments and which is not inhibited by failure. It is quite evident that progress is favoured by the assistance of adults which is always available. Nevertheless an infant who is left completely to itself learns without aid.

The infant acquires head control at 3 months, the ability to sit at 6 months, to crawl at 9 months, and walk with support at a year and independently at 15 months [6]. The range of normal is wide with a variation of two months on either side of the 'normal' being common.

Newborn Stepping

As the infant emerges from the neonatal period, it is able to control its head. Control of the head is the first stage of the development of walking. In general the development of motor control proceeds from rostral (i.e., the head) to caudal (i.e., the tail) and in the extremities from proximal to distal [7]. At this stage if the infant neonate is suspended over a supporting surface it takes 'steps' so-called 'newborn stepping' (see Figure 4.1). which comprises synchronous hip, knee, and

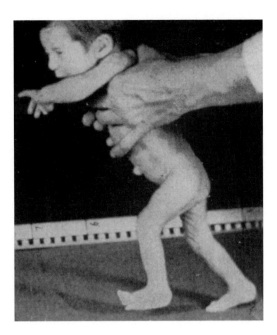

Figure 4.1. Stepping movements of a newborn. Frame of a film. (From Peiper A. Cerebral Function in Infancy and Childhood. Kluwer Academic Publishers Boston/Dordrecht London 1964.)

ankle flexion, followed by similar movements in extension [8]. The stepping movements of the newborn differ from a toddler walking in that only the legs are used: the other parts of the body do not participate. The legs can carry the weight of the body only for a few moments and the trunk cannot remain erect without support. If one were to let go the infant would immediately collapse. The newborn strides with slightly flexed hips and knees just as a toddler, that is, a child who has achieved independent walking but not yet achieved mature gait. These stepping movements have no temporal relationship to the child's mastery of walking. This phenomenon disappears in the second month of life, whereas walking starts towards the end of the first year [5].

Newborn stepping probably represents a spinal cord-mediated pattern of motor activation. Growth of the infant during the first year with relatively greater increases in mass than muscle strength probably explains why this phenomenon disappears in the erect position, whereas supine kicking persists.

At about ten months of age the child stands on bow legs held apart for balance, bent hips and knees, and a curved lower back [9]. Most reports of attempted gait analysis in children during supported walking have noted considerable inter- and intrasubject variability [10]. At first the child leans slightly forward and, to prevent falling, instinctively moves one leg forward ('the tottering biped' described by Earnest Hooton, a famous Harvard anthropologist).The child goes on so fast that it almost becomes a kind of run that it cannot stop, ending in a collision with the furniture or a fall. Thus a child seems to run before he/she can walk, because slower movement requires better balance; it has better dynamic than static balance [9]. The hip and knee are held in a greater degree of flexion throughout the gait cycle than is seen in the adult. The excessive flexion is most noticeable at the hip, giving the child the appearance of 'high stepping'. Initial contact with the ground is most often with a flat foot.

At the start of independent walking, the toddler steps with a wide base, holds the arms away from the body with the elbows extended and walks in a staccato manner. There is no reciprocal arm swing. The foot and ankle are held in exaggerated dorsiflexion during the stance phase (see Figure 4.2). Heel strike is absent as is the natural heel–toe progression. During the swing phase there is diminished dorsiflexion, and a relative foot drop. There is external rotation of the hips throughout the cycle, which requires circumduction to clear the foot during the swing phase. The width of the base gradually diminishes. Movements become smoother, reciprocal arm swing begins, and an adult pattern of walking emerges. Maturation of gait occurs rapidly. This can be judged by the duration of single

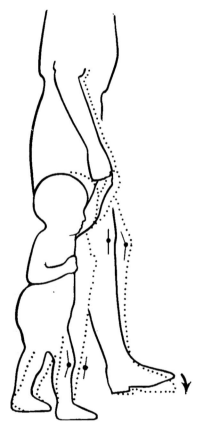

Figure 4.2. Diagram illustrating difference in knee and ankle positions of a normal child and a normal adult at the onset of weight bearing (solid line) and following the onset of weight bearing (dotted line). (Reprinted with permission from Statham L, Murray MP. Early walking patterns of normal children. Clin Orthop Relat Res. 1971;79:8–24.)

limb stance, walking velocity, cadence, step length, and the ratio of pelvic span (body width at anterior superior iliac spines) to ankle spread (the distance between the centres of left and right ankles during double support time) [11]. Most of these features can be observed in the clinic. It is more difficult to differentiate between step length, cadence, and walking velocity, but two observers with a stop watch can measure walking velocity and cadence and calculate step length (see Figures 4.3 and 4.4).

Gait

In adults about 38% of the gait cycle is spent in single limb stance. In one-year-olds the single limb stance is 32% of the cycle. Values approximating adult values are achieved by three and a half years [2]. The speed of a child increases with independent walking. In Statham and Murray's study [10] the increase in speed could be explained by an increase in cadence from 107 steps/min in supported walking to 158 steps/min in independent walking. The walking pattern of a nor-

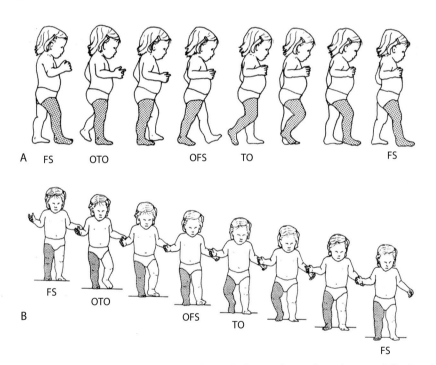

Figure 4.3. (A) Gait of one-year-old girl. Tracings of individual movie frames throughout one full gait cycle. The individual movie frames coincide with significant gait events. The cycle begins with right foot strike on the left and ends with foot strike of the same foot on the right. (B) Frontal view: FS, foot-strike; OTO, opposite toe-off; OFS, opposite foot strike; and TO, toe-off. (Reprinted with permission from Gait Disorders in Childhood and Adolescence, Sutherland DH, Lippincott Williams & Wilkins, 1984.)

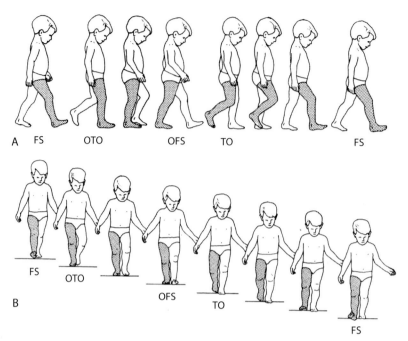

Figure 4.4. (A) Three-year-old normal gait pattern shows vigorous gait, reciprocal arm swing, well-developed heel strike, and smooth movements which differ only from an adult. (B) Frontal view with abbreviations as in Figure 4.3. (Reprinted with permission from Gait Disorders in Childhood and Adolescence, Sutherland DH, Lippincott Williams & Wilkins, 1984.)

mal three-year-old child resembles mature gait except that until around seven years old the child still has a higher cadence and walking velocity.

According to Wheelwright et al. [12] gait in normal children is not necessarily symmetrical. As a rule, left and right values were found to differ from one another by as much as eight to ten percent in any one individual. The mean ratio (left:right) of most variables was between 0.99 and 1.01 (a mean discrepancy of one percent) The asymmetry in the double support intervals was much greater (approximately nine percent) with a definite bias between the two sides: the double support time following the left stride was significantly shorter than the right ($p < 0.001$). A similar bias existed for both step length ($p < 0.01$) and swing time ($p < 0.05$), and again the discrepancy for these parameters was only one percent.

Todd et al. [13] (Figure 4.5) found that the relationship between stride length and walking speed was well represented by a parabola. A similar parabolic relationship was found between stride length and height. By four years the interrelationship between time/distance parameters is fixed, although stride length and walking velocity continue to increase with increasing leg length. It is interesting that the legs contribute only 37% of the total height of a one-year-old compared to 48% in the adult [7].

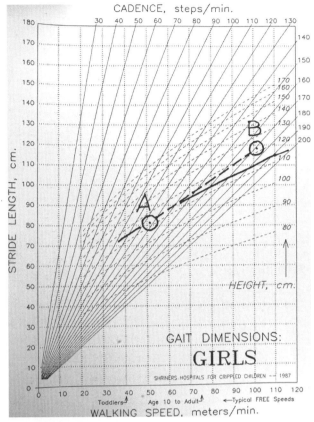

Figure 4.5. This represents the relationship between stride length and walking speed in girls. The data that are plotted are for a normal six-year-old girl whose height was 114 centimetres. The solid line which represents the normal parameters for height, is drawn on the chart for reference. (Reprinted with permission from Todd FN, Lamoreux LW, Skinner SR, et al. Variations in the gait of normal children. A graph applicable to the documentation of abnormalities. J Bone Joint Surg Am. 1989;71(2):196-204. © The Journal of Bone and Joint Surgery, Inc.) A = stride length, B = cadence.

Running

By the age of two most children can run. The child begins by running in a straight line. During play in the preschool years there is an increasing demand for the ability to change direction quickly to dodge and stop abruptly. Gradually the skill of running improves not only in terms of the ability to run in variable patterns but on different surfaces and terrain [14].

Centre of Gravity

In children the centre of gravity of the whole body is first found at about the level of the eleventh thoracic vertebra, just anterior to the vertebral column where the inferior vena cava enters the abdomen through the diaphragm; with maturation it descends to its adult level anterior to the second piece of the sacrum. The position of the centre of gravity can be estimated as 55% of the total height, measured from the soles of the feet [15].

The vertical displacement of the centre of gravity is a vital feature of body mechanics. In human gait the vertical displacement of the centre of gravity attempts to mimic the wheel by minimising the displacement and tracing the trajectory as a low sinusoidal curve to save energy. It is interesting to note that chimpanzees move their centre of gravity in the same manner as humans; it is high during the single-stance phase and low during the double-stance phase. Chimpanzees adopt this type of walking as early as two years of age. In the young animal standing upright the hip and knee joints are flexed more than in older infants and juveniles, just as in humans [16] (see Figure 4.6).

Changes in the Limbs

The position of the limbs in the foetus is one of flexion. The hips are flexed and externally rotated. The knees are flexed with internal rotation of the tibia and fibula. The ankles are often dorsiflexed with the feet internally rotated or supinated. The axis of the ankle joint is about 10 degrees externally rotated with

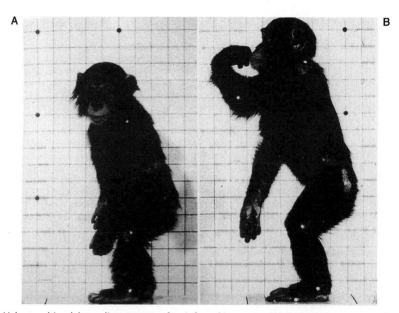

Figure 4.6. Voluntary bipedal standing posture of an infant chimpanzee (A) at two years two months of age; (B) At three years six months of age. The hind limb joints are more extended at the older age. (Reprinted from Kimura T. Centre of gravity of the body during the ontogeny of chimpanzee bipedal walking. Folia Primatol. 1996;66(1–4):126–36, with permission from S. Karger AG, Basel.)

reference to the axis of the knee. At birth the femoral neck is anteverted with respect to the femoral condyles. Once walking begins this angle is considerably reduced. With growth, remodelling produces an additional 12 to 15 degrees of external rotation of the hip over the first eight years [7].

The Foot

In the infant before walking has begun, there are traces of a prehensile great toe. Humphry in 1858 [17] wrote 'watch the movements in an infants foot, as yet unshod are considerably freer than your own; especially you will observe there is a power of separating the great toe from the others and approximating it to them.' This movement is almost always lost in the adult who continuously wears shoes and never goes barefoot (see Figure 4.7).

At birth and in infancy the sole of the foot appears flat because of the presence of a large sole pad which consists of 'fat enmeshed in extremely dense fibrous tissue' as observed by Wood-Jones [18]. However, as far as the bony and cartilaginous elements of the foot are concerned, the arches are present as soon as these elements take their definitive forms in foetal development. The sole of the foot is flat because the sole pad masks the arched arrangement of the underlying bones. The relative size of the sole pad reduces as the child grows.

The development of the longitudinal arch has been studied by Rose et al. [19] and Staheli et al. [20] in normal infants and children. Footprints were taken of children and measured. In Staheli's series metatarsal width, arch width, and width in the middle of the heel were recorded. From these measurements the ratios of arch width to metatarsal width, and arch width to heel width were calculated. The mean ratio of arch width to heel width is 1.27 in the child under six months; it decreases rapidly to 0.75 and then levels off throughout the rest of childhood.

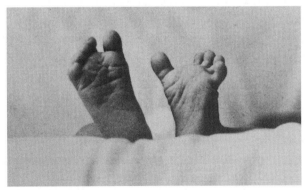

Figure 4.7. Showing the prehensile movements of the toes of an infant. (Reprinted from Susanne Szasz, 1954. Nouvelles Images Ltd., London.)

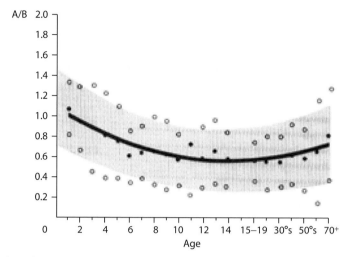

Figure 4.8. To show the mean value of the arch index and two standard deviations for each of 21 age groups. The solid line shows the mean changes with age; the shaded area the normal ranges. The actual values for each group are represented by solid circles for the mean and open circles for two standard deviations. (Reprinted with permission from Staheli LT, Chew DE, Corbett M. The longitudinal arch. A survey of eight hundred and eighty-two feet in normal children and adults. J Bone Joint Surg Am. 1987 Mar;69(3):426–8. © The Journal of Bone and Joint Surgery, Inc.)

The decreasing ratio of arch to heel width probably corresponds to the development of the arch and the reduction in size of the sole pad. In young children the standard deviations are large, indicating wide variation (see Figure 4.8). The average ratio of heel to total foot length changed little in a series of 20 children studied longitudinally by Anderson et al. [21]. The foot grows in harmony with the body as whole, rather than the lower extremity of which it is a part; the length from heel to toe maintained the same relationship to the length from heel to head at all ages during which the foot was increasing in size. Interference with the growth centres of the foot, whether by pathology or surgery, would have proportionately less deforming effect on the final length of the foot than would similar injuries to the growth centre of the femur and tibia. In general, the early adolescent spurt in the rate of growth of the foot preceded that in the long bones and stature by 6 to 18 months. The growth spurt of the foot is an early sign of the onset of puberty. At birth the foot is 40% of its final size. At the end of growth it represents 15% of the standing height in both boys and girls [22]. Anderson et al. give 16% with a range of less than 2%.

In a group of 125 children 11 to 14 months of age who were followed for four years by Gould et al. [23] at the initial examination all the apparently toddlers had flat feet. Arches developed regardless of the footwear worn.

Common Variations Which Disappear with Growth

Metatarsus adductus is the most common foot deformity [6]. It is not usually noted at birth but becomes increasingly obvious between 6 and 12 months. The foot is plantigrade and the heel neutral or slightly valgus with a convex lateral border and an increased separation between the great and second toes. Medial deviation of the great toe, or hallux varus, is accentuated on weight bearing. The forefoot deformity is at the level of the tarso–metatarsal junction. It is thought to be a result of the intrauterine position and almost always resolves spontaneously [24]. In intrauterine life the foot is minimally ossified and is readily affected by postural stress. The deformity may be exaggerated by sleeping in the prone position.

With growth femoral anteversion declines from about 30 degrees at birth to about 10 degrees at maturity. The tibia rotates laterally from about 5 degrees at birth to a mean of 15 degrees at maturity. White children are maximally bow-legged at 6 months and progress toward approximately neutral angles (zero degrees) at 18 months of age. The greatest mean knock-knee was 8 degrees at 4 years, followed by a gradual decrease to a mean of less than 6 degrees at 11 years [25].

Mechanical Work in Walking

Inman et al. [26] suggest that the human body integrates the motions of the various segments and controls the activity of the muscles, so that the metabolic energy required for a given distance walked is reduced to a minimum.

Walking in all animals (as in humans) involves an alternating transfer between gravitational-potential energy and kinetic energy within each stride as it takes place like a pendulum [27]. Kinetic energy is highest when potential energy is lowest and *vice versa*. This transfer is greatest at intermediate speeds and can account for up to 70% of the total energy changes taking place within a stride leaving only 30% to be supplied by muscles. When we walk on the flat the knee angle is 160 to 180 degrees for most of the stance phase. This allows walking with little activity in the muscles related to the knee. Another consequence is that the hip must rise and fall, describing an arc of a circle during the part of stance phase in which the foot is flat on the ground. This tends to make the potential energy fluctuations during a step balance the kinetic energy fluctuations [28]. The force exerted on the ground tends to remain in line with the leg throughout the step. If the force is aligned with the leg and the length of the leg remains constant, no work is done and potential and kinetic energy must balance.

Bound Feet

The now historical practice where the feet of young girls were deliberately deformed by binding indicates the plasticity of growing bones and is the opposite of standard treatment for deformities such as club foot. Miltner in 1937 [29] published an authoritative description of the technique and its effects. It is not known for certain when the practice started but it continued for about ten centuries in China until the establishment of the Chinese Republic in 1912 when the government was able to introduce effective legislation against the practice and end the seclusion and limited activity of women. In addition, the Mongolian pigtail which had been worn by the Chinese since 1644 ceased to be compulsory.

The process of binding which was mainly used in the upper class because poor women had to be able to work in the fields, was started sometime between four and eight years of age by the mother and was continued throughout the life of the individual. Two to four strips of cotton cloth or silk (in the wealthy) about three to five feet in length and two to three inches in width were used. Following repeated manipulations and bandaging over about a year it was possible to push the four lateral toes (sometimes with fractures) against the sole with marked narrowing of the forefoot. During the next two to three years the second stage of manipulation and binding was vigorously carried out.

After each treatment the feet were held in the new position with bandages applied in a figure-of-eight manner. Once the desired shape and size had been achieved the various layers of bandage were sewn together to act as a substitute for a cast. This was changed at intervals of several months. By the age of 11 or 12 the girl had acquired the art of applying her own bandages. Unless performed with gentle or experienced hands the process was associated with great pain and discomfort.

The anatomical effects can be seen in Figures 4.9A, B. Posture and gait were affected [30]. It was similar to walking on high heels. The legs were wasted but the thighs in contrast looked large, which made the women appear more voluptuous to the male Chinese observer.

If the feet were bound to a very small size (three to four inches in length) walking and running were grossly restricted. Chinese poets often referred to the three-inch golden lily. The curved pointed form of the feet was called the crescent and the shoes worn called bow-shoes. If bound to a moderate size (five to six inches in length) the woman was better able to cope.

Today the fashion of wearing high heels with pointed toes is the modern equivalent of how in the search for fashion women are still prepared to tolerate discomfort and risk future problems with their feet.

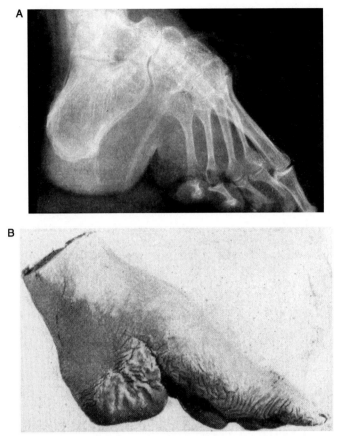

Figure 4.9. (A) Lateral radiograph of Chinese bound foot. (Reprinted with permission from Miltner LJ .Chinese bound foot. Bone Joint Surg. 1937;314–319. © The Journal of Bone and Joint Surgery, Inc.) (B) The external appearance of a bound foot.

Summary

The immature child grows and develops over a three to four year period, to be able to walk upright confidently. Clark and Phillips [31] pointed out that the task of walking is difficult as the propulsive forces are potentially destabilising (to a system that in its adult form is supported on only one leg for 80% of the walking cycle). The infant manages this problem quite simply by reducing this proportion to 40% and thus spending 60% of the gait cycle with both feet firmly on the ground. The result of this landbound approach, although assuring a measure of upright stability, affects forward propulsion (i.e., stride, velocity). The infant walker moves forward very slowly even in relative terms, at about half of the rate of adults, taking 'baby steps'. Nevertheless after two to three months of walking practice almost all the variables of gait are at least at the level of the 12-month walker. Once stable, progress is rapid.

References

1. Robinson RJ, Tizard JPM. The central nervous system in the new-born. *Brit Med Bull*. 1966; 22: 49–55.
2. Sutherland D, Olsen RA, Biden EN, Wyatt MP. *The Development of Mature Walking*. Oxford: Mac Keith Press; Blackwell Scientific; 1988: Chapter 11.
3. Morrell P, Norton WT. Myelin. *Sci Am*. 1980; 242: 74–89.
4. Forssberg H. A developmental model of human locomotion. In: Grillner S, Steiner PSG, Stuart DG, Forssberg H, Herman RM, eds. *Neurobiology of Vertebrate Locomotion*. Basingstoke, Hampshire: Macmillan; 1986: 486.
5. Peiper A. *Cerebral Function in Infancy and Childhood*. Translation of 3d revised German edition by Nagler B and Nagler H. London: Pitman Medical; 1996: 222.
6. Staheli LT. *Practice of Paediatric Orthopaedics*. Philadelphia: Lippincott, Williams & Wilkins; 2001: 9.
7. Skinner S.. Development of gait. In: Rose J, Gamble JG, eds. *Human Walking*. 2d edition. Baltimore, MD: Williams and Wilkins; 1994: Chapter 6
8. Farmer SE. Key factors in the development of lower limb co-ordination: Implications for the acquisition of walking in children with cerebral palsy. *Disability Rehab*. 2003; 25: 807–816.
9. Holle B. *Motor Development in Children Normal and Retarded*. Oxford: Blackwell Scientific; 1976: 28.
10. Statham L, Murray MP. Early walking pattern of normal children. *Clin Orthopaed Related Res*. 1971; 79: 8–23.
11. Sutherland DH, Olshen R, Cooper L, Woo SL. The development of mature gait. *J Bone Joint Surg*. 1980; 62A: 336–353.
12. Wheelwright EF, Minns RA, Law HT, Elton RA. *Develop Med Child Neuro*. 1993; 35: 102–113.
13. Todd FN, Lamoreux L, Skinner SR, Johanson MS, Helen R St, Moren SA, Ashley RK. Variations in the gait of normal children. *J Bone Joint Surg*. 1989; 71A: 196–204.
14. Wicksrom RL. *Fundamental Motor Patterns*. 2d ed. Philadelphia: Lea and Febiger; 1977: 37.
15. Black E. *Orthopaedic Management in Cerebral Palsy*. London: Mac Keith; 1987: 37.
16. Kimura T. Centre of gravity of the body during the ontogeny of chimpanzee bipedal walking. *Folio Primatol*. 1996; 66: 126–136.
17. Humphry GM. *The Human Foot and the Human Hand*. London: Macmillan; 1861: 84.
18. Wood Jones F. *Structure and Function as Seen in the Foot*. London: Balliere Tindall and Cox; 1994: 65.
19. Rose GK, Walton EA, Marshall T. The diagnosis of flat foot in the child. *J Bone Joint Surg*. 1985; 67B: 71–78.
20. Staheli LT, Chew DE, Corbett M. The longitudinal arch. *J Bone Joint Surg*. 1987; 69A: 426–428.
21. Anderson M, Blais M, Green WT. Growth of the normal foot during childhood and adolescence. *Am J Phys Anthropol*. 1956;14, 287–308.
22. Dimeglio A. *Growth of the Foot in Flatfoot and Forefoot Deformities*. Epeldegui T, ed. Madrid: A Madrid Vincente; 1995: 65.
23. Gould N, Moreland M, Alverez R, Trevino S, Fenwick J. Development of child's arch. *Foot Ankle Int*. 1988; 9: 241–245.
24. Rushforth GF. The natural history of hooked forefoot. *J Bone Joint Surg*. 1978; 60B: 530–532.
25. Heath CH, Shaheli RT. Normal limits of knee angle in white children – genu varum and genu valgum. *J Paediatric Orthopaed*. 1993; 13: 259–262.
26. Inman VT, Ralston HI, Todd F. *Human Walking*. Baltimore, MD:Williams & Wilkins; 1981: 3.
27. Cavagna GA, Heglund NC, Taylor CR. Mechanical work in terrestial locomotion: two basic mechanisms for minimizing energy expenditure. *Am J Physiol*. 1977; 233: R243–R261.
28. Alexander McNeill R. Human locomotion. In: Jones S, Martin R, Pilbeam D, eds. *The Cambridge Encyclopaedia of Human Evolution*. Cambridge: Cambridge University Press; 1992: Chapter 2.9.
29. Miltner LJ. Bound feet in China. *J Bone Joint Surg*.1937; xix: 314–319.
30. Chew MBK. Chinese bound foot. *Radiography*. 1973; xxxix: 39–42.
31. Clark JE, Phillips SJ.. A longitudinal study of intralimb co-ordination in the first year of independent walking. *Child* Develop. 1993; 64: 1143–1157.

5
The Measurement of Footprints (Pedobarography)

It happened one day about noon, going towards my boat, I was exceedingly surprised with the print of a man's naked foot on the shore, which was very plain to be seen in the sand. I stood like one thunderstruck, or as if I had seen an apparition, for there was exactly the very print of a foot, toes, heel and every part of a foot.

Daniel Defoe [1]

The human footprint is unique (see Figure 5.1). According to Wood-Jones it is the most distinctly human part of the whole anatomical make-up. Robinson Crusoe was quite sure there was another person on the island when he saw the footprint of the man, Friday. Similarly this was applied to the interpretation of the first record of bipedal walking preserved in cemented lava at Laeotoli in Tanzania; these footprints are direct evidence for hominins walking on two legs (see Chapter 2).

As pointed out by Lord Kelvin (William Thomson 1824–1907), the famous physicist, to measure is to know, 'I often say that when you can measure what you are speaking about and express it in numbers you know something about it; but when you cannot measure it, when you cannot express it in numbers your knowledge is of a meagre and unsatisfactory kind' [2].

This chapter deals with the development of methods of measurement of the pressure beneath the weight-bearing foot and how it affects our understanding of the function of the foot.

Measurement of the pressure beneath the foot is a specialised form of gait analysis which allows a study of the distribution of pressure across the sole throughout the stance phase. Simple measures of gait – cadence (i.e., the number of steps taken in a given time), stride length, and walking speed – can be based on measurements of length and time and were described by the Weber brothers (see Chapter 3). More sophisticated methods are necessary for mechanical analysis. The first graphic records of gait were made by Etienne Jules Marey (1830–1904), a leading figure of nineteenth century science, and his student Georges Carlet. These were based on Marey's earlier pneumatic transducers and consisted of an inner tube placed in the thick rubber sole of a shoe. When the foot made contact with the ground the inner chamber was compressed and actuated a lever via a pneumatic tube. The lever produced a recording on smoked paper fastened to a rotating drum. Marey and Carlet used this system to describe the different phases of gait and to record the duration of steps, the single and double support periods, and the swing phase. They also measured foot pressure. Their relatively simple apparatus allowed them to study not only walking but running and jumping. They could time the phases of single and double support during walking [3].

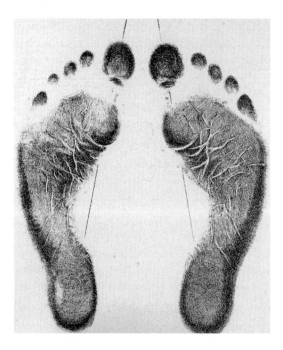

Figure 5.1. Impressions of the soles of an 11-year-old boy taken with printer's ink. The awkward look of a single sole print is not apparent when the two are seen together, the curves round the toes running into each other gracefully. The line, known as Meyer's line, is seen to run through the centre of the heel and along the midline of the great toe. It was thought to mark the principal line of action in the foot. (Reprinted from Ellis [38, Fig. 20].)

An attempt to study the distribution of foot pressure was made by Beeley in 1882 [4]. He had his subjects step on a thin sack filled with plaster of Paris. He thought that those portions of the foot carrying the greatest weight would make the deepest impressions. However, this method records the shape of the foot not the pressure. It is interesting to note that in 1890 Arthur Conan Doyle in his book, *The Tale of Four*, allows Sherlock Holmes to say, 'Here is my monograph upon the tracing of footsteps, with some remarks upon the uses of plaster of Paris as a preserver of impresses.' He was clearly up to date for the time [5].

Subsequently, many different techniques have been used and with the advent of microelectronics have now reached an advanced stage of development. Small computers allow data to be rapidly acquired and displayed. The development of pressure measurement systems has been stimulated by the potential for computer-aided design (CAD) and computer-aided manufacture (CAM) for the production of footwear and insoles [6].

Lord [7] has carried out an extensive historical survey of the development of methods for measuring the pressure beneath the sole of the foot. She has pointed out that there are three approaches to the development of foot ground pressure, between the sole of the bare foot and the ground, between the plantar surface of the foot and inside of the shoe, and between the sole of the shoe and the ground. Lord et al. stressed that when making measurements beneath the feet it is important to distinguish between force, a push or pull applied to a body (mass × acceleration) measured in newtons, and pressure (force per unit area) measured in pascals which is one newton per square meter or more commonly stated in kilopascals as the pascal is inconveniently small. Major contributions were made by Schwartz [8], Elftman [9], and Morton [10]. Instantaneous pressure distributions were recorded by Elftman for the first time in 1934. He used a mat with rubber pyramids on one side, which was laid on a glass plate. By stepping on the mat the contact area of the pyramids was increased. A 16 mm cine film (72 frames/s) of the illuminated glass plate produced a record of instantaneous pressure. This chapter deals only with the techniques that are in common use at present and the measurement of normal function.

Force Plate

A force plate consists of a load-sensitive surface set into a walkway, which measures the changing forces imposed on it during the period of foot contact. As advances were made in electronics more complex techniques have been developed. According to Hutton and Stokes [11], a group at the University of California (1947) and Cunningham and Brown (1952) both described a force plate, which used strain gauges as the transducing elements. A typical force plate in current use consists of a rigid rectangular plate about 50 × 30 cm set into the floor of a walkway and supported near each corner by load cells. Vertical, longitudinal, and transverse forces and also torque can be measured separately [12]. It is also possible to derive the centre of load, the point on the force plate at which the force exerted between the foot and the ground can be considered to act [13].

Elftman and Manter in 1934 were the first to describe a method by means of which the distribution of pressure at any instant could be recorded cinematographically as a pattern of dots, the area of the dot varying with the pressure being exerted [29]. By the method of moments it was possible by extensive calculation to determine the position of a resultant force having the same effect as the various discrete pressures recorded. The position of this resultant must lie on the axis of the foot, if the axis as usually considered represents the line of functional symmetry. In other words, one can refer to a plane of symmetry, and say that the resultant lies in the line of intersection of this line and the horizontal. Nowadays this centre pressure line can readily be calculated by a computer and printed out in relation to a footprint using computerised techniques of foot pressure measurement (see Figure 5.2). It is also interesting to see how it varies from the human to the foot of a great ape (Figure 5.19) [30], where it passes from the centre of the heel to the middle toe instead of, as in the human, to the second toe.

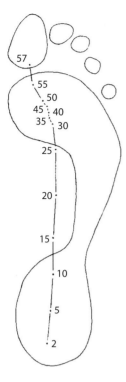

Figure 5.2. The pathway of the centre of load, the point through which the load on the foot can be considered to act during the stance phase of walking expressed as percentages of the walking cycle. Each point was derived by finding the centre of load of the longitudinal and corresponding transverse patterns at successive instants. (Reprinted from Hutton and Stokes [11].)

An essential feature that has to be considered in the design of a force plate is the frequency response of the system. This is a measure of how fast and with what accuracy the system will respond to abrupt changes in load. To accurately transduce the forces imposed on it, a load-measuring system must have a low natural frequency which is substantially higher than any of the applied frequencies [14]. The elastic response of the deformation of the material plays a major role.

Pressure Transducers

The use of pressure transducers provides a convenient method of studying the forces on selected areas of the foot. One particular advantage over other methods is that they can be worn inside shoes and are thus useful for studies on footwear and insoles. However, there are a number of problems associated with the interpretation of the records generated by transducers. The sole of the foot is irregular in contour and varies in compliance from the relatively unyielding region under the metatarsal heads to the softer areas under the midfoot. As a result the force transmitted across the region of the foot in contact with the floor changes markedly with small changes in position. It is important to know how a transducer, which may have a large pressure-sensing area, summates forces that vary from point to point across the surface. A further difficulty that is inherent in sampling only a few points under the sole of the foot is the problem of inferring the pressure elsewhere on the foot. A large number of small transducers are required to integrate pressure values over a specific area to derive the total force transmitted [11]. Reproducibility is also a problem as it is difficult to be sure that the transducer is always positioned in the same place as previously used.

Modified Force Plates

An apparatus to give a dynamic visual display of force distributions on the plantar surface of the foot was developed by Chodera and Lord [15]. It consisted of a plastic foil placed on a glass plate illuminated through its edge on which a subject can walk or stand, thus pressing the plastic foil into contact with the glass. The contact areas between the glass and the plastic foil reflect light downward and the intensity of reflected light varies with the applied pressure. The image produced by the foot was recorded with a television camera and displayed using a contour plot or a colour scale to indicate pressure levels [16]. Clinical applications of this system are described by Betts et al. [17] and it is commercially available as the dynamic pedobarograph, a term first introduced by Chodera (see Figures 5.3 to 5.5).

Dhanendran et al. [18] subdivided a force plate into 12 independent strips, each recording the vertical load against a base of time. The strips could be

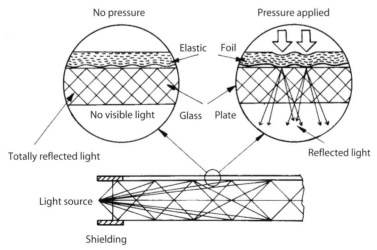

Figure 5.3. To show the principles of the optical dynamic pedobarograph. Plastic foil when deformed by weight bearing alters the distribution of light within an illuminated box.

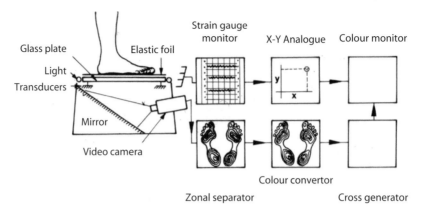

Figure 5.4. A side-view of the optical pedobarograph, showing the videocamera and a diagram of the final picture.

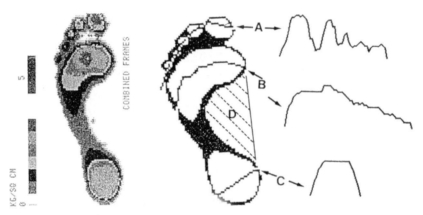

Figure 5.5. Combined frames (summary picture) in black and white from an optical pedobarograph of a foot bearing eight and showing distribution of the pressure at the toes (A), metatarsal heads (B), heel (C), and (D) the arch during the stance phase.

oriented either transversely or longitudinally to the direction of walking and their output used to generate the longitudinal and transverse load profiles. This was followed by a further development of a force plate subdivided into 128 squares of 15 × 15 mm each, which recorded vertical load. Data were collected and analysed by computer. Ten normal subjects were recorded walking over this machine, and also over the dynamic pedobarograph and the Harris and Beath mat (see Figures 5.6 to 5.8). This mat was developed as part of an investigation of the feet of Canadian soldiers mentioned in Chapter 3.

It consists of a commercially-produced rubber mat, which is covered with fine ridges at three levels; to use it, a glass plate and water-soluble printers' ink are required. A small quantity of ink is rolled out on the glass plate until it is of

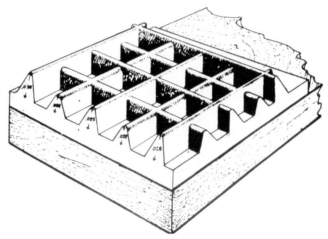

Figure 5.6. A close-up of Harris and Beath mat showing the ridges of varying size arranged orthogonally in two directions.

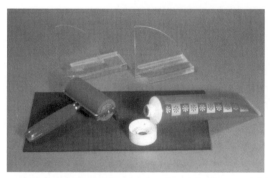

Figure 5.7. The equipment to make measurements on a Harris and Berth mat: soluble printer's ink, and a rubber printing roller. Two set squares are used to project the prominent edges of the malleolli downward onto the recording paper.

uniform thickness. Ink is applied to the surface of the mat with the roller. Walking or standing on a sheet of plain paper placed on the mat produces an imprint of the foot showing the area in contact with the ground and also a two-tone indication of pressure. The parts of the foot exerting the least pressure print only the highest ridges to produce a light-coloured image whereas greater pressure prints the deeper ridges as well, giving a darker image. Very high pressure can be distinguished by all the ridges being completely printed. It is a slightly messy technique! The study [19] concluded that the dynamic pedobarograph was not as accurate as the modified force plate but that good resolution made it a clinically useful tool, because clinicians familiar with pattern recognition as in electrocardiograms and radiographs would find this method of recording foot

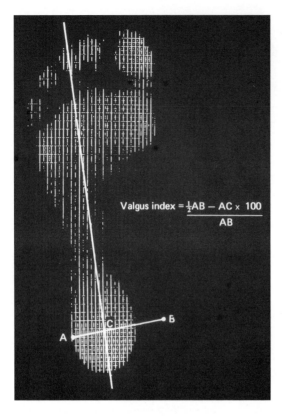

$$\text{Valgus index} = \frac{\frac{1}{2}AB - AC \times 100}{AB}$$

Figure 5.8. An example of a footprint on a Harris and Beath mat with the formula to estimate a Valgus Index as suggested by Rose et al. (Reprinted with permission from Rose et al. [39].)

pressures of more practical use than precise numbers. The only advantage of the Harris and Beath mat is that it is relatively cheap, but it is difficult and laborious for absolute measurements.

A variety of force plates has appeared on the market. One in common use is based on the work of Nicol and Hennig [20] and uses capacitance transducers as the sensory elements. It has been developed by Novel Gmbh in Munich (the system is commercially available as EMED). The individual transducers can have a small surface area, thus giving good spatial resolution. A capacitance transducer (Figure 5.9) consists of two plates made of a conducting material separated by a nonconducting or insulating layer, a dielectric. The transducer stores an electrical charge and the two plates are compressed when force is applied, causing the distance between the two plates to decrease. As the distance between the plates decreases, the capacitance increases and the resulting change in voltage is measured. The EMED system platforms are available in different sizes and with various local resolutions. The variables of measurement are pressure (recorded in newton/cm^2), time in seconds, and site of pressure (in *X/Y* co-ordinates; Figure 5.10). There is also a system for in-shoe measurement which is very useful for testing

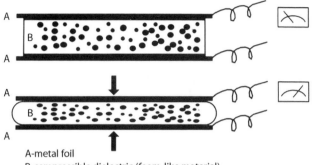

A-metal foil
B-compressible dielectric (foam-like material)

Figure 5.9. Diagram of a capacitance transducer: A, metal foil; B, compressible dielectric (foil-like material). (Copyright © 1991 by the American Orthopaedic Foot and Ankle Society, Inc., originally published in Foot & Ankle International, Alexander JJ, Chao EY, Johnson KA. The assessment of dynamic foot-to-ground contact forces and plantar pressure distribution: a review of the evolution of current techniques and clinical applications. Foot Ankle. 1990 Dec;11(3):152–67, reproduced here with permission.)

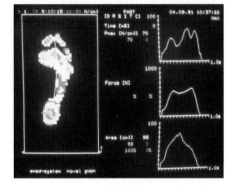

Figure 5.10. Typical recording from EMED apparatus with summary of pressures on the foot. The area taking the load, the total, and peak pressure can be seen on the right side. (Reprinted with permission from Rose GK, Welton EA, Marshall T. The diagnosis of flat foot in the child. J Bone Joint Surg Br. 1985 Jan;67(1):71–8.)

the effects of orthotics, shoe research and design, and biomechanics in sport (Figure 5.11).

The metric configuration of the sensors provides for identification of each sensor for calibration. All sensors are simultaneously loaded in steps and a specific calibration curve for each sensor is calculated. Only calibrated values (using SI units) are displayed. The calibration can be verified by the user. The number of sensors per square centimetre varies from 1 to 9 depending on the requirements of the user. For foot pressures 4 per cm^2 is common. A large variety of EMED systems is available. They differ in size, number of sensors, resolution, and sampling frequency.

A comparison of the EMED and the dynamic pedobarograph has been carried out [21]. Both studies examined 100 normal adult Caucasian volunteers with ten men and ten women in each of the following age groups 20–29, 30–39, 40–49, 50–59, and 60 plus. Comparison of the results from the two methods showed that

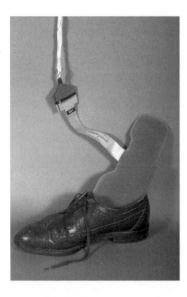

Figure 5.11. The insole for in-shoe measurement (Pedar-x System)

the median peak pressures demonstrated similar patterns with the highest pressure in the forefoot under the second/third metatarsal heads and the toes taking gradually reduced pressure from the first to the fifth toe. The EMED system showed higher peak pressures than the dynamic pedobarograph under the heel, the medial four metatarsal heads, and the great toe, but lower peak pressures and shorter contact times under the lateral four toes. With about 12 different systems available on the market standardisation for comparison between systems is very important [22].

Laboratory Practice

There is a problem with the units for measurement of pressure. The SI unit is the pascal (Pa), that is, 1 newton per square metre. This is a very small unit of pressure and for practical purposes the unit K Pa is used. Americans use pounds per square inch (psi), EMED systems use newtons per square centimetre (N/cm^2), and other systems quote kilograms per square centimetre (kg/cm^2). For standardisation, pressure mats need to be placed within walkways, sunk into a space beneath the floor, and not left standing free. Walkways should be rigid and when above floor level, support the mat on a rigid base. There should always be sufficient space to allow at least three steps before and after the mat and preferably more. It is best if the mat is invisible. In some laboratories pressures are measured after the first step as it is easy to perform and less time consuming.

Measurements of the first step have been reported as giving pressures seven to ten percent less than free walking. As the speed of walking influences the consistency of the measurement of plantar pressures in some studies, walking speed has been controlled by a metronome. Free walking at the subject's normal pace is the most desirable approach. As callus on the plantar skin increases the foot pressure it is best for studies to be carried out after chiropody. The optimum number of trials before the measurements are taken is at least three [23]. It must also be remembered that measurement of pressure distribution when standing does not correlate well with dynamic loads during walking. Measurement of both peak pressure and pressure time integral are of importance. High transient pressure may be less harmful than a moderate sustained pressure and this is a useful measurement to note. It is inevitable from the variations in specifications for each system that each laboratory must establish its own range of normality.

The reliability of foot pressure measurement has been tested using the EMED F System. Ten volunteers had 25 walks recorded at three different speeds. Coefficients of reliability calculated for 1 to 25 walks showed that a good measure of reliability was achieved using one measurement for most force/pressure variables but when the mean result of three or more walks was used reliability was excellent. Measurements related to time were more variable than the total force, the peak pressure, and the area. The total force and peak pressure were also shown to increase with increasing speed, but this was not true for all sites on the foot (see Figures 5.12 and 5.13). It is clear that a mean of several walks is more reliable than a single measurement; at least three measurements should be made for research projects which aim to compare groups of several different subjects [24].

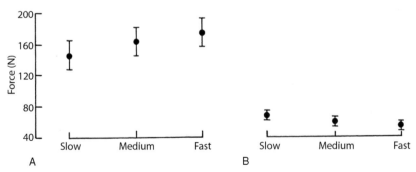

Figure 5.12. Plots of the mean and its 95% confidence interval for force under (A) the first and (B) the fifth metatarsal heads showing the increase in force with speed for one and the decrease for the other. (Reprinted from Hughes J, Pratt L, Linge K, et al. Reliability of pressure measurements: the EMED F system. Clinical Biomechanics 1991;6:14–18, © 1991, with permission from Elsevier.)

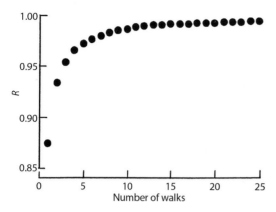

Figure 5.13. Graph of the coefficient of reliability plotted for 1–25 walks for total force at medium speed. (Reprinted from Hughes J, Pratt L, Linge K, et al. Reliability of pressure measurements: the EMED F system. Clinical Biomechanics 1991;6:14–18, © 1991, with permission from Elsevier.)

Loading of the Normal Foot

Measurements of foot pressure have helped to improve our understanding of the functions of the foot. The use of the toes has been described in Chapter 3. The development of weight bearing has been studied in the child.

Using an EMED system with a mat with two sensors/cms sq a comparative study was carried out on a group of children: seven boys and eight girls aged between 14 and 32 months. A group of 111 adults was used for comparison. The children showed a substantial reduction in peak pressures in all the related areas (medial heel, lateral heel, midfoot region, first metatarsal head, third metatarsal head, fifth metatarsal head, and hallux) with the exception of the midfoot area. This was thought to be due to the softer structure and increased fat of the infant foot and by a 1.5 times higher body weight to foot contact area ratio in the adults. The adults load a smaller area in relation to their body weight.

There was a difference in mechanics between adults and children. High relative loads under the midfoot region and a fairly even distribution under all the metatarsal heads reveal that the longitudinal arch has not yet fully developed in the infant. A comparison of walking and running patterns in children showed a higher loading of the first ray with reduced stress on the lateral aspect of the forefoot during running. With growth the relative load under the midfoot decreases, and load beneath the third and fifth metatarsal heads increases. Within a few months a rapid development of the growing foot to an adult pattern is observed [25] (see Figure 5.14). In another study by Hennig and Rosenbaum of 125 children between six to ten years of age, compared to 111 adults [26], considerably lower peak pressures were again found in the children. A shift of load to the medial side of the forefoot was observed in the older children. The reduced loading of the first metatarsal head in the younger children was explained by valgus knees with pronation of the foot and reduced stability of the first ray. Genu valgum (see Chapter 4) is a common variation in children that in most cases disappeared by the age of seven. The fact that there was no reduction in pressures under the lon-

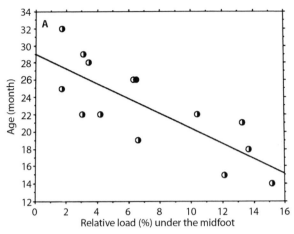

Figure 5.14. A correlation between age and relative load under the midfoot region in children. (Copyright © 1991 by the American Orthopaedic Foot and Ankle Society, Inc., originally published in Foot & Ankle International, Hennig EM, Rosenbaum D. Pressure distribution patterns under the feet of children in comparison with adults. Foot Ankle. 1991 Apr;11(5):306–11, reproduced here with permission.)

gitudinal arch suggests that the development of the longitudinal arch is complete before the age of six years. Contrary to the findings in adults, body weight was found to have a major influence on the magnitude of the pressures under the feet in school-aged children. There were no differences in peak pressure or relative load patterns between boys and girls.

Assessment of Foot-pressure Patterns from a Pedobarograph Using Techniques of Imaging Analysis

The analysis of the pressure distribution under the foot using a pedobarograph has been well documented [27]. Quantitative information about pressure patterns is digitally recorded and the peak pressures under prescribed areas may be calculated. Descriptions of the resulting pressure patterns as a whole have been subjective and often lengthy, even for a single footstep. An analysis can be made by classifying the overall dynamic foot pressure patterns. The information necessary to produce such patterns is transferred from the recording microcomputer to a mainframe computer and thence to an image analysis system. A software programme has been developed to automatically find specific regions of the foot on the pressure image and graphically display patterns of pressure across the forefoot (28). The following groups were found in a series of 160 normals [12] (see Figure 5.15).

Medial pattern with highest load medially	16%
Medial/central pattern – equal loading across first and second metatarsal heads	14%

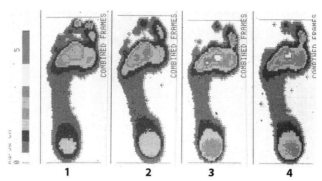

Figure 5.15. The four patterns of loading on the forefoot: 1, Medial; 2, medial central; 3, central; 4, lateral.

Central, those feet with highest loading centrally under the second
  or third metatarsal heads   60%
Lateral pattern – feet with central and lateral loading   10%

They illustrate the variability of gait but also confirm that central loading under the second and third metatarsal heads is very common.

The Effect of High and Low Heels

The effect of walking with high heels on the distribution of plantar foot pressure was investigated in ten healthy female volunteers. It was performed with the Micro-EMED (Novel Gmbh) in-shoe pressure measurement system with capacitance sensors. It has a homogeneous distribution of 85 sensors with local resolution of one sensor per 2 cm^2. It is 2 mm thick and flexible enough to adjust to the shape of the shoe. The shod foot measurements were taken while the subjects walked on a treadmill at a regulated speed of 4 km/h for at least five min. It was found that high-heel shoes increased the load on the forefoot and relieved it on the hind foot. The load passed toward the medial forefoot and the great toe. The lateral side of the forefoot showed a decrease in contact area, reduced forces, and peak pressures. The medial side of the forefoot had a higher force-time and pressure time integral. The duration of contact time in the medial forefoot suggested that the area was loaded throughout the stance phase. The findings may well be related to the development of hallux valgus and hallux rigidus [31].

The Effect of Obesity on Patterns of Foot Pressure

An investigation of 13 obese children and 13 nonobese controls examined the effects of obesity on the distribution of plantar pressures. The mini-EMED (Novel Gmbh, Munich) system was used for measurement. It was found that temporary increases of mass by loading the subjects with an additional 20% of body mass resulted in increased static and dynamic plantar pressures but no significant change to the structure of the feet of prepubescent children. However, long-term increases of mass associated with obesity appeared to flatten the medial longitudinal arch of the children as confirmed by an increased area of foot contact with the ground. Whether this is permanent or reversible by loss of mass is unclear [32] (Figure 5.16) A similar result was found in adults of both sexes. The greatest effect was found under the longitudinal arch and the metatarsal heads [33]. These findings are relevant to the problem of lack of physical activity and obesity in childhood.

Shear Forces

During normal walking the sole of the foot is subjected to vertical and horizontal or shear forces. Shear may be subdivided into both longitudinal and transverse components. Measurement of all these forces is changed under pathological conditions. It has been shown, for instance, that in the diabetic foot high vertical pressures are associated with the presence of neuropathic ulcers and are thought to be an important aetiological factor in their formation. It has been suggested that high shear stresses are also important in the development of such ulcers. Despite the number of systems available for measurement of vertical forces, there has been a dearth of systems designed to measure shear stresses on the sole of the foot. A shear transducer small enough to be worn comfortably under a normal foot linked to a microcomputer data logger was developed in Liverpool [34].

Preliminary studies showed that the shear forces measured in a group of ten normal volunteers who walked barefoot on a treadmill were bidirectional. Forward shear was found under the heel on heel strike and backward shear under the

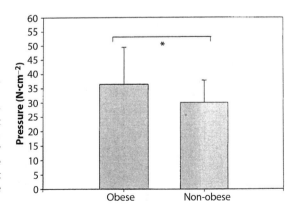

Figure 5.16. Forefoot dynamic pressure (mean I sd) derived for obese (*n* = 13) and nonobese (*n* = 13) children. *indicates a significant difference between the subject groups. (Reproduced with permission from Dowling AM, Steele JR, Baur LA. Does obesity influence foot structure and plantar pressure in pre-pubescent children? Int J Obes Relat Metab Disord. 2001;25(6):845–52, © Nature Publishing group.)

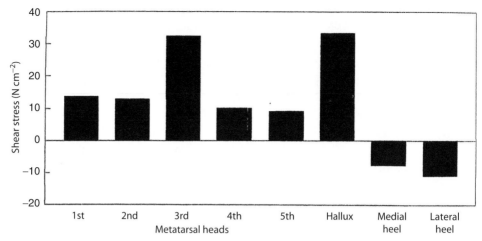

Figure 5.17. Measurement of shear stress in the forefoot taken with the Liverpool shear force low profile transducer.

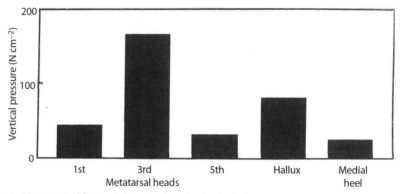

Figure 5.18. Mean vertical forces at the same five sites in the foot.

metatarsal heads on toe-off. The higher mean shear stresses and vertical pressures were found under the great toe and third metatarsal heads. Shear stress was approximately 30% of the value of the vertical pressures with a range of 19.5 to 40.9%. Using linear regression, shear stresses were found to be highly significantly correlated with vertical pressures at all the five sites on the feet that were compared (see Figures 5.17 and 5.18). It is possible that the concept of a total force load on the foot that includes both vertical and horizontal components may be important.

Plantar Pressures in the Great Apes

Elftman and Manter [35] first compared the distribution of plantar pressures in humans and the chimpanzee. An understanding of how the foot of a great ape functions is of value in the interpretation of the transition of the prehensile foot to the plantigrade foot of humans. Wunderlich and Ford [36] studied two male seven-year-old male chimpanzees (51 and 58 kg). Dynamic plantar pressure distribution was collected using an EMED-SF platform mounted in a wooden runway. The results showed a distinct difference in load distribution during bipedal

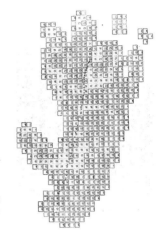

Figure 5.19. Footprint of orangutan showing wide separation of hallux from lesser toes and a relatively straight centre of pressure line passing from the heel to the middle toe.

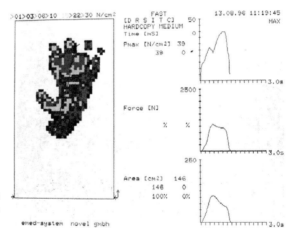

Figure 5.20. Summary footprint with details of maximum pressure force and area over time.

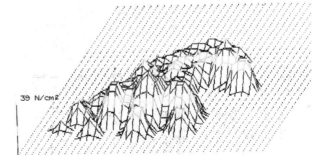

Figure 5.21. The same footprint illustrated in three dimensions.

compared with quadrupedal walking.The chimpanzee when walking upright differs from the human in that there are high pressures in the midfoot region, relatively long hindfoot and midfoot contact times, and low forefoot loading. It resembles walking in young children [25] (see Figures 5.19 through 5.21).

Vereecke et al. [37] studied the walking of bonobos, or pygmy chimpanzees (*Pan paniscus*) using force plates and pressure mats (RScan International). They found that there was a midtarsal break as a consequence of a flexible midfoot. Because of this the heel can be lifted before the midfoot leaves the ground. They observed a distinct region of pressure under the lateral midfoot, which remained after heel-off. The heel and lateral midfoot typically touch down simultaneously at initial contact with the ground. There is no clear peak pressure under the heel, and the heel occasionally touches down in the second half of the stance phase. Pressure distributions under the heel, medial midfoot, metatarsal heads, and hallux are relatively constant throughout the stance phase. At toe-off there is pressure under the lateral toes, but there is no peak pressure under the hallux. These findings are a marked contrast to those in the human foot where, because of a longitudinal arch, there is no midfoot contact at all; instead there is evidence of a well-marked heel strike and pressure under the metatarsals and toes.

Summary

The development of methods of measurement of plantar foot pressures has been described. They have proved to be of great importance in gait analysis. It adds quantitative precision to the study of the weight-bearing foot. Because of the variety of techniques available there is need for standardisation so that results from different laboratories can be compared. The EMED system is so far the most efficient and accurate. At present the role of foot pressure measurement is almost entirely academic. Although it has been used for extensive study of important clinical problems such as diabetes and rheumatoid arthritis, as well as design of insoles, it has not yet been integrated into daily clinical practice to become part of routine assessment comparable to the ECG in cardiology. Nevertheless it is invaluable for comparison of the patients' clinical assessment and as a method of comparison of the pre- and postoperative state to confirm whether the purpose of the operation has been achieved. In the future this should be possible with small portable easily-operated apparatus available in an outpatient clinic, and it should be possible to measure both vertical and shear forces at the same time.

References

1. Defoe D. *Robinson Crusoe*. New York: A Signet Classic. The New American Library; London: The New English Library Limited; 1960. 152.

2. Thompson S. *The Life of William Thomson Baron Kelvin of Langs* in two volumes. Vol II. London: Macmillan;1912:792

3. Bouisset S, Marley E-J. On when motion biomechanics emerged as a science. In: Cappozo A., Marchetti M., Tosi V. eds. *Biolocomotion: A Century of Research Using Moving Pictures*. Promograph. Rome; 1992: Chapter 5, 77–79.

4. Beeley F. Zur Mechanik des Stehens v. Langebecks, *Archive fur Chirurgie*. 1882; xxvii: 459–471.

5. Doyle A.C. *The Sign of Four*. London: Penguin Classics. Penguin Books; 2001: 8.

6. Lord M., Reynolds DP, Hughes JR. Foot pressure measurement: A review of clinical findings. J Biomed Eng. 1986; 8: 283–294.

7. Lord M. Foot pressure measurement: A review of methodology. *J Biomed Eng*. 1981; 3: 91–99.

8. Schwartz RP, Heath AL. The pneumographic method of recording gait. *J Bone Joint Surg*. 1932; 14: 783–793.

9. Elftman HO. A cinematic study of the distribution of pressure in the human foot. *Anat Rec*. 1934; 59: 481–490.

10. Morton DJ. *The Human Foot*. New York: Columbia University Press; 1934: 155.

11. Hutton W, Stokes TAF. Biomechanics of the foot. In: Klenerman L, ed. *The Foot and Its Disorders*. Oxford: Blackwell Scientific; 1991: Chapter 2, 12.

12. Stokes IAF, Stott JRR, Hutton WC. Force distributions under the foot. *Biomech Eng*. 1974; 9: 140–143.

13. Grundy M, Blackburn TPA, McCleish D, Smidt I. An investigation of the centres of pressure under the foot while walking. *J Bone Joint Surg*. 1975; 75B: 98–103.

14. Marsden JP, Montgomery SR. An analysis of the dynamic characteristics of a force plate. *Meas Control*. 1972; 5: 102–106.

15. Chodera J.D., Lord M. Pedobarographic foot pressure measurements and their applications. In: Kennedi RM, Paul JR, Hughes J, eds. *Disability*. London: Macmillan; 1979:173

16. Betts RP, Duckworth T. A device for measuring plantar pressures under the sole of the foot. *Eng Med. Ins Mech En*g. 1978; 7: 223–225.

17. Betts RP, Duckworth T, Austin IG. Critical light reflection at a plastic/glass interface and its application of foot pressure movements. *J Med Eng Technol*. 1980; 4: 136–142.

18. Dhanendran M, Hutton WC, Paker Y. The distribution of forces under the human foot – An on line measuring system. *Meas Control*. 1978; 11: 261–264.

19. Hughes J, Kriss S, Klenerman L. A clinician's view of foot pressure: A comparison of three different methods of measurement. *Foot Ankle*. 1987; 7: 277–283.

20. Nicol K, Hennig EM. A capacitance type measuring system for exterior biomechanics. *J Hum Move Stud*. 1981; 7: 83–86.

21. Hughes J, Clark P, Linge K, Klenerman L. A comparison of two studies of the pressure distribution under the feet of normal subjects using different equipment. *Foot Ankle*. 1993; 14: 514–519.

22. Barnett S, Faculty of Health and Social Care, Foot Pressure Interest Group. University of West of England, Bristol. Personal communications.

23. Young M. Draft protocol guidelines. *Diabetic Foot*. 1988;1: 137–139.

24. Hughes J, Pratt L, Linge K, Clark P, Klenerman L. Reliability of pressure measurements. *Clin Biomech*. 1991; 6:14–18

25. Hennig EM, Rosenbaum D. Pressure distribution patterns under the feet of children in comparison with adults. *Foot Ankle*. 1991; 11: 306–311.

26. Hennig EM, Rosenbaum D. Plantar pressure distribution patterns of young school children in comparison to adults. *Foot Ankle Int*. 1994; 15: 35–40.

27. Betts RP, Franks CI, Duckworth T, Burke J. Static and dynamic foot pressure measurements in clinical orthopaedics. *Med Biolog Eng Comput*. 1980; 18: 674–84.

28. Hughes J, Jagoe JR, Klenerman L. Assessment of foot pressure patterns from a pedobarograph using image analysis techniques. *Proc Physiol Soc J Physiol*. 1987; 384; 7.

29. Elftman H., Manter J.T. The axis of the human foot. *Science*. 1934; LXXX: 484.
30. Elftman H, Manter J, Chimpanzee and human feet in bipedal walking. *Am J Phys Anthropol*. 1935; xx: 70–79.
31. Nyska M, McCabe C, Linge K, Klenerman L. Plantar foot pressures during treadmill walking with high-heel and low-heel shoes. *Foot Ankle Int*. 1996; 17: 662–666.
32. Dowling AM, Steele JR, Baur LA. Does obesity influence foot structure and plantar pressure patterns in pre-pubescent children. *Int J Obesity Related Disord*. 2001; 25: 845–852.
33. Hills AP, Hennig EM, McDonald M, Bar-Or O. Plantar pressure differences between obese and non-obese adults: A biomedical analysis. *Int J Obesity*. 2001; 25: 1674–1679.
34. Laing P, Deogan H, Cozley D, Cogley D, Hammond P, Klenerman L. Development of low profile Liverpool shear transducer. *Clin Phys Physiol Meas*. 1992; 13: 115–124.
35. Elftman H, Manter J. Chimpanzee and human feet in bipedal walking. *Am J Phys Anthropol*. 1935; xx: 67–79.
36. Wunderlich RE, Ford KR. Plantar pressure distribution during bipedal and quadripedal walking in the chimpanzee (*Pan troglodytes*). In: Proceedings of EMED Scientific Meeting 2–6 August, 2000: 19.
37. Vereecke D'Aout K, De Clerq D, Van Elsacker L, Aerts P. Dynamic plantar pressure distribution during terrestial locomotion of bonobos (*Pan paniscus*) *Am J Phys Anthropol*. 2003; 120: 373–383.
38. Ellis TS. *The Human Foot*. London: J. & A. Churchill; xxx1 1899.
39. Rose GK et al. The diagnosis of flat foot in the child. *J Bone Joint Surg*. 1985; 67(1): 71–88.
40. Alexander IJ, Chao EY, Johnson KA. The assessment of dynamic foot-to-ground contact forces and plantar pressure distribution. *Foot Ankle*. 1991; 11: 152–165.9.

6
The Foot in Action

This chapter deals with some of the many varieties of human activity in which the function of the foot is tested to the extreme and used with maximal skill, such as running, ballet dancing, kicking, and for swimming, tightrope, and fire-walking. These various skills are due to central neurological control. In contrast in microgravity the role of the foot is changed with consequences that are described.

The Armless or the Foot as a Hand

In the armless the foot can be developed to be used almost as skilfully as the hand. When the absence of limbs is congenital, the child has no experience of a normal body and does not miss anything in the first years of life. This is well illustrated by a patient of LK's who was a victim of thalidomide, but was self-sufficient, could feed himself, and write. A better-known example is Herman Unthan who deserves an important place among the records of the handicapped. His autobiography records his varied and interesting experiences of someone without arms. He learned to write, play several musical instruments, and swim, and he earned his living while travelling alone over two continents [1]. There is also The Association of Mouth and Foot Painting Artists with about 650 members in 60 countries throughout the world with high artistic standards (see Figure 6.1).

Footedness

Footedness, that is, using one foot in preference to the other is related to handedness, Most right-handers are right-footed and left-handers are left-footed. The footedness of professional soccer players has been assessed by how often they touch the ball with the right or left foot. Most use their preferred foot about 85% of the time, and almost none use each foot the same number of times. In other words, even professional footballers cannot use both feet equally well. Like the rest of the population, 20% of footballers are left-footed, a percentage substantially higher than 10% or so for left-handed people. Some right-handers are 'cross-lateral,' writing with their right hand and kicking with their left foot [2]. This bias to the right is connected to the functioning of the left and right cerebral hemispheres [3] which has probably been present since

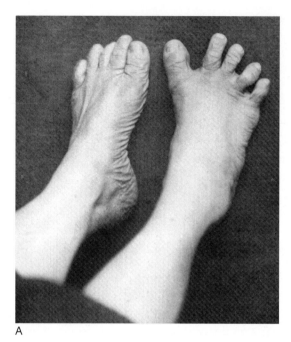

A

Figure 6.1. (A) To show the mobility in the toes of an armless man.

the early stages of human evolution for it is claimed that some of the earliest stone artefacts show signs of a preference for being made by a right-handed stone knapper.

Starosta [4] in an extensive analysis of shots at goal during World Cup and other high-level competitions showed that the most successful players shot for goal with both left and right feet. He concluded that the development of the ability to kick with either foot should be part of the preparation for all skilled players.

Running

Sir Roger Bannister, the first man to run the mile in less in less than four minutes, describes how he felt when as a boy he ran on a beach: 'The earth seemed almost to move with me. I was running now, and a fresh rhythm entered my body. No longer conscious of my movement I discovered a new unity with nature. I had found a new source of power and beauty, a source I never dreamt existed' [5].

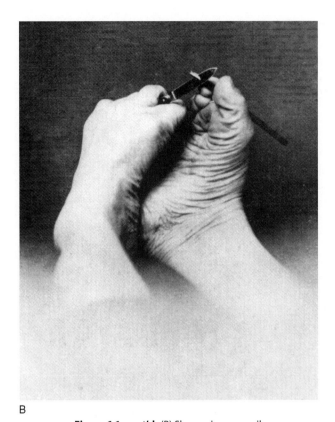

B

Figure 6.1. cont'd (B) Sharpening a pencil.

The natural movement of some runners will be apparent to anyone who has an eye for rhythm and flow: the variety of styles and forms has to be seen to be believed. Some are better suited to running faster than others. It does not mean that they are better people, but their physiological blueprint enables them to start out with a physical advantage in that particular movement.

David Hemery, winner of 400 metres hurdles at the 1968 Mexico Olympics in world record time [6]

When speed is not a factor, people walk. They run to go faster. The same basic mechanisms occur in the lower limbs and feet in running and walking. The duty factor (i.e., the fraction of total time each foot is on the ground) is greater than 0.5 for walking and less than 0.5 for running [7]. The essential difference between the two is that during running both feet are off the ground for part of the stride. The body is propelled through space wthout support from either leg. This situation reduced to the minimum support produces the version of running commonly known as jogging. This simple form of running is characterised by a slow pace, a

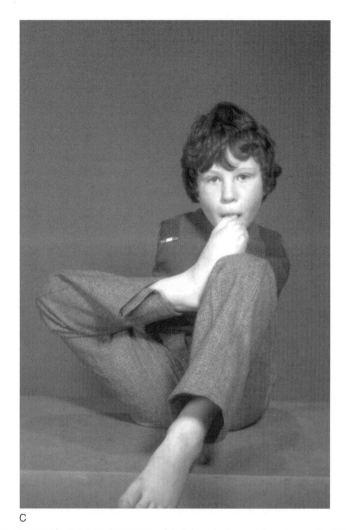

Figure 6.1. cont'd (C) An armless victim of thalidomide showing how he can feed himself.

short stride, and a bouncing motion. Running at increasingly greater velocities leads progressively to sprinting, the ultimate version of running that is designed for speed; sprinting involves a fast pace, a long stride, and minimal bounce [8].

There is an important difference between sprinting and distance running because in the latter, the foot first touches the ground with the heel. In the sprinter, the ball of the foot touches down first, so that the forward movement of the thigh is slowed but not reversed and the knee flexes approximately 10 degrees. In long distance running, as the heel strikes the ground first, there is a slight reversal in the direction of the thigh and knee flexion of about 25 degrees. In a study at the University of Saskatchewan, in the sprint the stance phase lasted

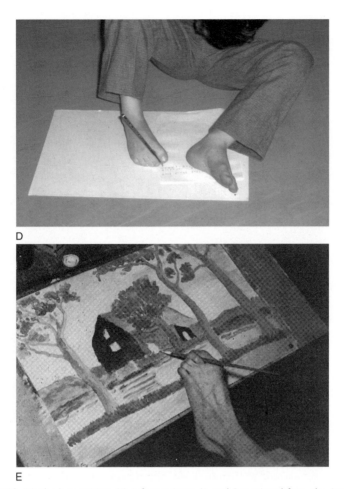

Figure 6.1. cont'd (D) The boy writing. (E) A foot painter. (A and B reprinted from the Armless Fiddler by C.H. Unthan, George Allen, and Unwin, London 1935, with permission of the Wellcome Library, London.)

on average 19% of the time of the stride, whereas in the long distance runner it lasted 28% [9]. In the sprint the limbs go through relatively shorter but quicker angular movements which provide great thrust while more time is spent in the unsupported phase and less in the support phase (see Figure 6.2).

Humans will choose to walk rather than run at speeds up to 2.5 m/s. Above this speed the energy required to walk exceeds that required to run. Humans as well as other animals tend naturally to adopt the most economical gait for a given speed so that the transition occurs at about this point [10].

In ancient times it was common to run barefoot and one only has to look at the paintings on 500 BCE Grecian vases to confirm this. Nowadays, although there have been famous exceptions, there is no good biomechanical reason to run

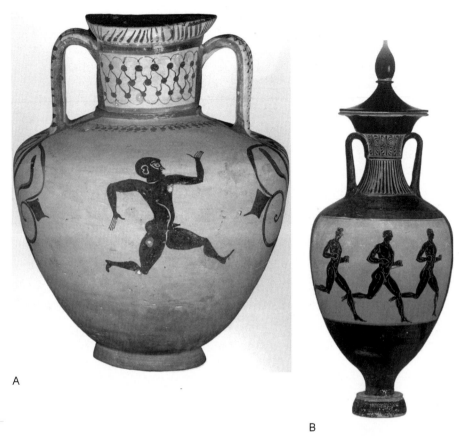

Figure 6.2. (A) A Greek amphora of about 550–525 BCE, showing the typical vigorous action of a sprinter. (B) Three long distance runners on a Panathenaic amphora of 333 BC. The body position differs markedly from (A). Olive oil was in the amphora which was decorated with a picture of the goddess Athena on one side and the contest at which the prize was won on the other. (Reprinted with permission. © Copyright The British Museum, London.)

barefoot. Abebe Bikila, who won the Olympic marathon in 1960 and Zola Budd, who ran for Britain in 1984 at Los Angeles are notable exceptions. Barefoot running minimises pronation. De Wit and De Clercq [11] studied the stance phase during both barefoot and shod running. They found that barefoot running is characterised by a significant larger external loading rate and a flatter foot placement at touchdown. The flatter foot placement correlates with lower peak heel pressures. Nevertheless, with asphalt and concrete pavements, icy roads, and broken glass, it is only the idealist who persists in running barefoot. The problem is to determine an acceptable degree of pronation. The running shoe industry has capitalised on the proposed association between injuries of the lower limb and the feet and has developed entire shoe lines based on the idea of providing control of the foot.

In his book, *Biomechanics of Running Shoes*, Nigg [12] discusses the forces in relation to running. The maximum vertical forces are about 2.5 times body weight, and there is no difference between running barefoot and running with shoes. The maximum active vertical forces in sprinting are about 3.6 times body weight. In general with the active forces, the vertical peaks double from walking to running and triple from walking to sprinting. The internal active forces (i.e., forces inside the human body) cannot be measured but they can be estimated with the help of a model of the body or parts of it. Dynamic forces in the ankle joint were estimated by Seirig and Arvikar [13]. The maximum forces during walking were 5.2 times body weight. During sprinting the forces are increased to 13 times body weight. Internal forces can easily be a multiple of the externally measured forces.

One of the fascinating questions in relation to running is the superior performance of Africans and people of African descent in some athletic events. The Kenyans and Ethiopians from East Africa are small and excel in middle and long distance running. In contrast the sprinters from West Africa and North America and the Caribbean countries tend to be bigger and stronger people. The success of the sprinters is due to their more powerful muscles, which can also probably contract at faster speeds. This is in contrast to the long distance runners who have the ability to work closer to their maximum effort for longer than matched non-African runners. They also have thin and elastic legs and seem to bounce over the ground [14].

According to McNeill Alexander [10] the reason that running is so much more efficient than might be expected seems to be that much of the energy is not designed to last. Some of it is converted to elastic strain energy. The mechanism is like a bouncing ball, which converts kinetic energy into elastic strain energy as it deforms and hits the ground, and which then makes the reverse mechanical conversion as it recoils and leaves the ground again. In running, most of the elastic strain is stored in tendons [10] such as tendo Achillis and the tendons and ligaments supporting the medial longitudinal arch of the foot. Tendon is a remarkably good elastic material in that 93% of the work done stretching is returned in the elastic recoil. It can stretch by only 8% of its length before breaking, so long tendons are needed to make effective springs.

Working in South Africa, Wells [15] studied differences between the feet of the Bushman, Bantu, and white populations. He identified differences in the longitudinal arch. The medial arch is lower in the Bantu and Bushman than in the Europeans, the anterior limb being concavoconvex or even concave, not convex as in Europeans. In the two African groups, he suggested that there was additional support provided by peroneus longus and in part by the thickened superficial fascia of the sole. He also observed that at the level of the tarsometatarsal joint in Europeans, the lateral cuneiform projects distal to the other tarsal bones, thus locking the base of the second metatarsal as in a mortice. In the Bushman and

Bantu this arrangement is not present. Whether these anatomical differences are related to function is unknown as there have been no comparative studies of the modern human weight-bearing foot.

Most research on the evolution of human locomotion has focused on walking. Humans are mediocre runners. Even elite runners are comparatively slow, capable of sustaining maximum speeds of just over 10 metres per second for less than 15 seconds. However, although comparatively poor sprinters, they can perform endurance running covering many kilometres for long periods using aerobic metabolism. No primates other than humans are capable of endurance running. Although endurance running is now confined to sport it may have given humans an evolutionary edge, according to Bramble and Lieberman in a recent review [16].

Ballet Dancing

> To most balletgoers, the aristocratic foot of the dancer is the distinguishing feature of classical ballet. Strong and supple and as sensitive as a hand, the foot is used by the dancer in a manner that to the eye of the observer, departs distinctly from the ordinary mechanics of movement.
>   . . . Sensations relayed from the foot inform the rest of the body of the level of its support, its trajectory, its orientation in space and countless subtleties that are reflected instantly in every movement. It is no exaggeration to say that the qualities of a dancer's movement is directly related to the level of sensitivity in the use of the feet.
> Valerie Grieg [17]

These elegant descriptions encapsulate the role of the foot in ballet dancing, which is the acme of foot function. The grace and elegance of ballet has been beautifully portrayed by the French impressionist painter and sculptor Edgar Degas (1834–1917) in many works. Classical ballet is based on five positions of the feet and body from which the steps and movement of all ballet start and end. These five basic positions have one characteristic in common: external rotation of the hips or 'turnout' (see Figure 6.3A). This was first introduced as a theatrical adaptation of the fashionable fencer's stance. Turnout helps the dancer increase flexibility and balance while permitting the body to open outward toward the audience [18]. It is the cornerstone of correct ballet technique. It is not confined to the hip; it is the sum total of external rotation of the entire leg involving the hip, knee, ankle, and foot, but begins at the hip and then involves all the distal elements of the leg. Without proper turnout the dancer must constantly compensate which often wreaks havoc from the knee downward [19].

As a result of prolonged balletic activity, a pattern of cortical thickening occurs involving the shaft of the femur, tibia, fibula, and one or more of the first three

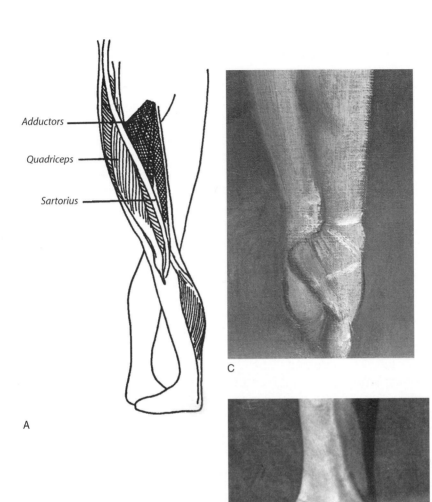

Adductors

Quadriceps

Sartorius

A

C

B

Figure 6.3. (A) Proper turnout must come from the hip down not from the feet up. (Drawing reproduced from Inside Ballet Technique: *Separating Fact from Fiction in the Ballet Class* by Valerie Grieg copyright © 1994 by Princeton Book Company, Publishers.) (B) The foot of Rudolf Nureyev en pointe, an unusual position for a male ballet dancer. (© Sally Soames, The Sunday Times, NI Syndication Limited, 1978.) (C) Close-up view of the feet of a ballet dancer en pointe, from the painting *Two Dancers on a Stage* by Edgar Degas. (The Samuel Courtauld Trust, Courtauld Institute of Art Gallery, London.)

metatarsal bones. The second metatarsal is most often involved and shows an increase in circumferential thickness resulting in a larger bone [20].

Female classical dancers dance *en pointe*. This technique is usually said to have been introduced by Marie Taglioni (1804–1884). It enabled her to appear ethereal and weightless and skim across the stage [21]. En pointe is the position of standing on the tips of the toes in specially made pointe shoes. The foot is in maximum plantarflexion or equinus and is in line with the shin (see Figures 6.3B, C). Men do not use pointe shoes as they usually dance on half pointe, which is the elevated position achieved by standing on tiptoes. A study with transducers to determine the relative pressures on the first and second toes and first metatarsophalangeal joint while dancing en pointe showed that the first ray always bore the most pressure irrespective of the length of the second toe. Pressures on the second toe varied as a function of toe length and spacing [22]. A study of nine ballet dancers standing en pointe was performed using a mould technique with alginate powder, which when hydrated solidifies to a mould in 30 to 60 seconds. These moulds showed three positions of the toes: (1) there was no crossing of the three medial toes; (2) there was crossing of the third toe behind the second; and (3) the hallux crossed partially across the front of the second toe [23]. For the best distribution of pressure on the forefoot the toes should be aligned side by side.

Ogilvie Harris et al. [24] examined 49 ballet dancers active in the National Ballet of Canada. Women with a second toe shorter than the hallux had the greatest daily foot comfort. Those with a second toe equal in length to the hallux had the lowest incidence of injuries to their feet and ankles. A second toe longer than the hallux was associated with the highest incidence of hallux rigidus. This study refuted the hypothesis that the ideal foot has a second toe equal in length to the hallux which is thought to allow a larger surface area to support the body weight when dancing en pointe.

When dancing en pointe the ballerina stands on her toes, which are only protected by the pointe shoe toe box. This protection is reduced when the toe box loses its structural integrity so it is essential that pointe shoes are replaced before they deteriorate. Most pointe shoes will fit either foot; there is usually no left or right. At the Royal Opera House in London the average allocation is ten pairs of ballet shoes per month [25]. The box of the shoe tightly encloses the toes so that the dancer's weight rests on an oval platform. The foot is supported under the arch by a stiff insole or shank. The shank has varying degrees of flexibility and the box may have different configurations

Albers et al. [26] showed by measurements on an EMED mat that simply wearing pointe shoes significantly increased the peak pressures acting through the foot. This was attributed to the fact that the pointe shoe is designed to provide stability and not to absorb or attenuate shock and there is also a reduction in the plantar surface area in contact with the ground.

Relevé, going to en pointe position from a plié (i.e., with knees flexed), showed peak pressures greater than pressures occurring while walking in pointe shoes or simply rising en pointe from a position with straight knees.

Modern, jazz, or ballroom dance and even some forms of folk dance share with ballet many similarities in the types of movements used [27].

The Foot in Microgravity

The structure of the foot has evolved so that it can respond to the force of gravity [28]. Because of the fundamental importance of dynamic gravitational loading, it is reasonable to expect that the skeleton is especially sensitive to changes in gravity. Changes in the strength of the gravitational field they do affect body mass, but weight. On the Moon and Mars our weight is 17 and 40%, respectively, of what it is on Earth, whereas on Jupiter it is estimated it would be 236%. It is difficult to maintain a normal walking pattern when the acceleration of gravity is reduced because of the imbalance between kinetic and potential energy [29]. Magaria and Cavagna [30] predicted the optimal speed of walking to be 1.8 km/h on the moon. They pointed out that when running on the moon the acceleration of the body at the start will be much less than on Earth. Skipping and hopping were the mode of locomotion preferred by members of the Apollo missions.

An astronaut in space is essentially weightless. This lack of weight is not because of lack of gravity but is rather due to a phenomenon called free fall; which means that the scale used to measure weight and the weight to be measured (the astronaut) are being identically accelerated by gravity, and as a result no weight is registered by the scale [31]. In space despite physical training regimes the bone loss that occurs as an adaptive process may result in skeletal damage after astronauts return to Earth. In-flight exercise training is a very important countermeasure. The types and amounts of exercise are still under debate. All Soviet space stations have treadmills. Soviet cosmonauts use a special elasticised suit, which provides passive stress on antigravity muscle groups of the legs and trunk. Elastic 'bungee cords' are used to secure the individual to the treadmill and provide simulated gravitational force [32]. Astronauts with the Skylab showed approximately four percent bone loss in the calcaneum as a result of the mechanical unloading of the bone over a six-month period [33].

Tightrope Walking

The most popular form of tightrope walking is the high-wire act where a taut springy wire is used to launch acrobatic tricks and phenomenal feats of balancing.

Slack wire, where the rope or wire hangs more loosely, is popular for juggling and clowning.

One way to view the high-wire act is to see the wire as an axis and the centre of mass or gravity of the performer as having the potential to begin to rotate about the wire. If the centre of gravity is not directly above the wire, the performer will rotate about the wire and, if corrective action is not taken, will fall. Tightrope artists often carry a balance pole that may be up to 12 m long and weigh up to 14 kg. This pole increases the rotational inertia of the artist and thus allows more time to move the centre of gravity back to the desired position directly over the wire. This effect can be magnified by making the pole as long as possible and weighting its ends. The pole helps balance by lowering the centre of gravity. It is possible to have such heavy weights attached to the end of a long drooping pole so that (theoretically) the centre of gravity of the performer/pole system is below the wire. In this case, it has been suggested the performer would require no more sense of balance than a person hanging from the wire but they do require considerably more courage [34].

Blondin, the pseudonym of Jean-Francois Gravelet (1824–1897) was a tightrope walker and acrobat who owed his celebrity and fortune to his feat of crossing Niagara Falls on a tightrope 1110 feet long and 160 feet above the water. He crossed the Falls a number of times, first in 1859, with different theatrical variations: blindfolded, in a sack, trundling a wheelbarrow, on stilts, carrying a man on his back, and sitting down midway to make and eat an omelette. In 1861 he appeared in London at the Crystal Palace and turned somersaults on stilts on a rope stretched across the transept 170 feet off the ground [35] (see Figure 6.4b).

One of the most dramatic and daring of recent tightrope performances was a high-wire performance by Philippe Petit, a young Frenchman who one night in 1974, secretly and illegally rigged a tightrope between the twin towers of the World Trade Centre. At daybreak he made eight crossings over the course of an hour, 110 floors up above ground level, wearing buffalo-skin soled slippers [36]. In *To Reach the Clouds* Pettit recommends that in order 'that the foot will feel the cable and not lend itself to accidental slips buffalo-hide slippers are recommended, though in rainy weather these should be replaced by slippers with rubber soles. But any unreinforced shoes with the main sole removed or even thick socks – several on each foot will do the job quite well' [37].

He states, 'the balancing pole is generally a wooden or metal tube with a diameter that allows easily handling. It is five to eight metres in length. Its weight varies according to the situation: the exercise balancing pole weighs twenty pounds; the balancing pole used in great crossings can be as heavy as fifty pounds.' He also stresses the need to practise barefoot. The wire passes between the great and second toe, crosses the foot along the whole length of the sole, and escapes behind the middle of the heel. One must be able to use the great and second toe to grip the wire and to hang on to it. 'This is the only way to avoid a slip during a Death Walk.' (See Figure 6.4A.)

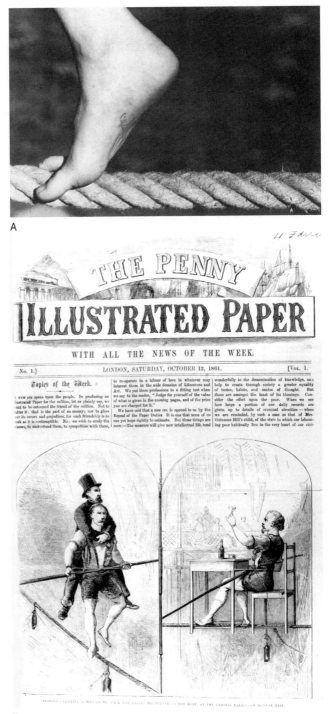

Figure 6.4. (A) Grasping the tightrope between the great and second toes to obtain a good hold. (Philippe Petit's right foot from *On the High Wire* by Philippe Petit. Random House New York 1985. Photograph by Thierry Orbach 1977.) (B) Blondin the famous tightrope walker crosses with a man on his back and also eating an omelette at leisure. (From *The Penny Illustrated Paper*, London, 12 October 1861, No. 1, Vol. 1. By permission of The British Library.)

Firewalking

Firewalking was practised in classical Greece and in ancient India and China. It still continues in many parts of the world, including India, Malaya, Japan, China, Fiji Islands, Tahiti, New Zealand, Mauritius, Bulgaria, and Spain. Many cultures incorporate firewalking into religious and mystical rituals. There are Hindu and Tibetan Buddhist firewalkers (see Figure 6.5). Firewalking takes several forms, the most common being the practice of walking swiftly over a layer of embers spread thinly along the bottom of a shallow trench.

Various explanations are offered as to the purpose of firewalking. Its performance is said sometimes to ensure a good harvest, other times to purify a person. Firewalkers believed that only those that lack faith will suffer injuries from fire, and the faithful are spared. Injuries from burns do occur but they seem on the whole, to be much less frequent than would be expected, especially as devotees do not apply any artificial preparation to the feet before the ordeal [39].

A number of theories have been proposed to explain the relative lack of injury to firewalkers. The dry wood coals used by many firewalkers conduct heat very

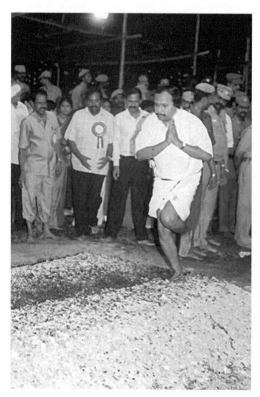

Figure 6.5. A firewalker at a Hindu festival. (Photograph courtesy of Professor S. Rajasekaran, Ganga Hospital, Coimbatore, India.)

poorly. The coal itself may be very hot but will not transfer heat to an object touching it. Wood is such a poor conductor of heat it is considered a good insulator. Any ash that builds up improves insulation. The coals are an uneven surface and the area of the foot touching the coals at any instant is small. Firewalkers do not spend very much time on the coals as they keep moving quickly.

Perception of pain is complex. Some people experience great pain without an apparent cause. Others suffer little or no pain, despite severe injury. Cognitive and emotional factors are important. A belief that one has control over the pain seems to reduce the level of pain. The following quotation indicates the state of mind of a firewalker.

> I ripped the shoes and socks from my feet and bounded on to the runway of fire. It was hot! It was very hot! Even as my mind shrieked at the insanity of what I was doing, my heart thrilled with exuberance, my body tingled with delight and I knew, I knew, my feet would not be burned. I half-laughed and half-shouted as I finished the walk. Before my mind had a chance even to demand that I check my soles, I made an about-face and again strode the coals. A part of me died that instant, another part of me was born. What died was a constricting belief system, and what was born was a sense of life's limitlessness.
>
> 'How? How is this possible?' I demanded when I finally inspected my unharmed soles.
>
> His companion replied, 'I don't know. I don't really care. What does it matter? There's no need for an explanation. It's possible and it's healthy. What else matters?'
>
> Tolly Burkhan [39]

Kicking

Kicking, like many of the skills in football, has been shown to develop from an early age. Children can kick a ball shortly after they are able to run, at about 18 months, but the movements are haphazard and barely recognisable as a pattern.

Wickstrom has defined kicking as 'an unique form of striking in which the foot has been used to impart force to a ball' [40]. This description refers to a variety of actions such as the instep kick, the punt which is when the ball is first held by the hands and then dropped onto the moving foot, the side-footed pass, the drop-kick when the ball is dropped on the ground and then kicked as it bounces, and the chip kick to lift the ball up into the air. Kicking occurs in all sports classified as football. The list includes Association football (soccer), rugby football, Gaelic football, and American football.

Wickstrom has separated the components of a mature kick into the following stages.

1. A preliminary forward step on the support leg to rotate the pelvis backward on the opposite side and to extend the thigh of the kicking leg
2. A forward swing on the kicking leg with simultaneous flexion at the hip and knee
3. Vigorous extension by the lower part of the kicking leg
4. A momentary cessation of the forward movement of the thigh and continued extension of the lower leg just before the foot contacts the ball
5. A forward swing of the opposite arm in reaction to the vigorous swing of the kicking leg

Novice adults are able to acquire kicking skills with relatively little practice [41].

Impact forces on the front of the ankle are of importance in understanding the development of the so-called 'footballer's ankle' where osteophytes grow out on the anterior margin of the tibia and the talus. This condition was described in detail by McMurray in 1950 [42] when he suggested that a tendency to traction on the capsular ligament occurs when the plantarflexed foot makes contact with ball on the anterior part of the ankle. Asami and Nolte 1995 [43] estimated a mean contact force of 1200 N and a peak force of 2400 N in professional footballers performing a maximal instep kick. Work from Holland based on arthroscopic findings has shown that the anterior capsule does not attach to bone at the site where the anterior talotibial spurs originate, but about 5 mm above the joint line. Osteophytes form on this nonweight-bearing cartilaginous rim of the tibia. It is likely that the damage from repeated microtrauma directly on the non-weight-bearing articular cartilage on the anterior edge of the articular surface of the tibia and likewise on the talus is the cause of the osteophytes [44].

Kicking skill begins to show signs of breaking down under the requirements of speed and accuracy [45]. Nevertheless as soccer is reputedly the most popular sport in the world, kicking remains the commonest skill related to the foot (see Figures 6.6 and 6.7).

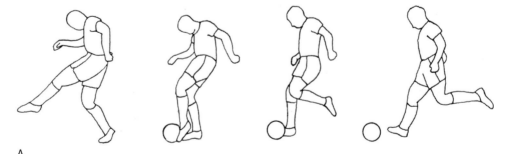

A

Figure 6.6. From right to left, the stages of the movements involved in a mature instep kick, showing the position of the supporting foot and corresponding body adjustments. (Modified with permission from Wickstrom [40].)

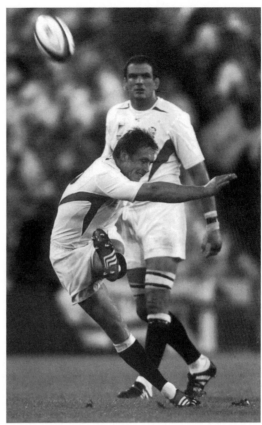

Figure 6.7. cont'd (B) A famous drop kick under pressure by Jonny Wilkinson which won the 2004 World Cup for England. (© Marc Aspland, The Sunday Times, NI Syndication Limited, 2003.)

B

SWIMMING

The legs and feet both contribute to the propulsive force of all four swimming strokes: front crawl, backstroke, breaststroke, and butterfly. However, propulsion for the kick requires a much greater output of energy compared to that derived from the arms.

The leg movements used are similar in all of the strokes except the breaststroke. There are two basic movements, an upward movement and downward movement known as the upbeat and downbeat. The downbeat is the propulsive phase in the front crawl and dolphin kicks. The upbeat is the propulsive phase of the backstroke flutter kick. Flexibility at the ankle joint with the capacity to point one's toes like a ballet dancer is a definite advantage (see Figure 6.8A, B). Loose ankles allow a supple weaving action. Foot size must be a factor and almost certainly contributes to the success of outstanding performers such as Ian Thorpe of Australia, a world record and Olympic champion front crawl swimmer who takes size 17 shoes [46].

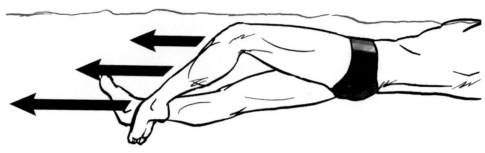

Propulsion during the upbeat of the backstroke flutter kick.

A

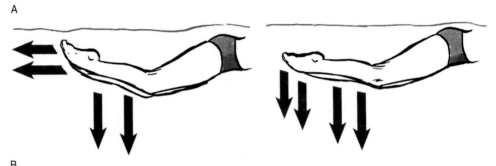

B

Figure 6.8. (A) The use of the foot in swimming backstroke. (From E.W. Maglischo, *Swimming Fastest*, page 175, figure 5.21. © 2003 by Ernest W. Maglischo. Reprinted with permission from Human Kinetics Publishers, Champaign, IL.) (B) The position of the feet in a dolphin kick. The more flexible the ankle, the more powerful is the propulsion as seen in (A), whereas in (B) the range is restricted and less effective. (From E.W. Maglischo, *Swimming Fastest*, page 87, figure 3.18. © 2003 by Ernest W. Maglischo. Reprinted with permission from Human Kinetics Publishers, Champaign, IL.)

References

1. Unthan C.H. *The Armless Fiddler*. London: George Allen and Unwin; 1935.
2. C. McManus. *Right Hand, Left Hand*. Great Britain: Weidenfeld and Nicolson; 2002: 152.
3. Annett M. The brain in left handedness. In: Jones S, Martin R, Pilbeam D, eds. *The Cambridge Encyclopaedia of Human Evolution*, Cambridge: Cambridge University Press; 1992: 122.
4. Starosta W. Symmetry and asymmetry in shooting demonstrated by elite soccer players. In: Reilly T, Lees A, Davids K, Murphy W, eds. *Science and Football*, London: E and F.N. Spon; 1988: 346–355.
5. Bannister R. *First Four Minutes*. London: Putman; 1955: 11.
6. Hemery D. *The Pursuit of Sporting Excellence*. London: Willow Books, Collins; 1986: 14.
7. Alexander R McNeill. Human locomotion. In: Jones S, Martin R, Pilbean D, eds. *Cambridge Encyclopaedia of Human Evolution,* Cambridge: Cambridge University Press; 80–85.
8. Wickstrom RL. *Fundamental Motor Patterns*. London: Henry Kimpston. 1977: 37.
9. Dagg A.I. *Running, Walking and Jumping*. London: Wykham; 1977: 49.
10. Alexander McNeill R. Walking and running. *Am* Sci. 1984; 72: 348–354.

11. De Wit WB., De Clercq D, Aerts P. Biomechanical analysis of the stance phase during barefoot running. *J Biomech*. 2000; 33: 269–278.
12. Nigg BM. Experimental techniques used in running research. In: Nigg BM, ed. *Biomechanics of Running Shoes*. Champaign, IL: Human Kinetics; 1986: 27–61.
13. Seireg A, Arvikar RJ. The prediction of muscular load sharing and joint surfaces in the lower extremities in walking. *J Biomech*. 1975; 8: 89,102.
14. (a) Noakes T. Professor, Department of Human Biology, University of Cape Town, personal communication. (b) Copetzer P, Noakes TD, Sanders B, Lambert MI, Bosch AN, Wiggins T, Dennis SC. Superior fatigue resistance of elite black runners. *J Appl Physiol*. 1993; 75: 1822–1827. (c) Weston AR, Karanigrick O, Smith A, Noakes TD, Myburg KH. African runners exhibit greater fatigue resistance, lower lactate accumulation and higher oxidative enzyme activity. *J Appl Physiol*. 1999; 86: 915–923.
15. Wells LH. The foot of the South African Native. *Am J Physl Anthropol*. 1931; XV: 186–287.
16. Bramble DM, Lieberman BE. Endurance running and the evolution of *Homo*. *Nature*. 2004; 432: 345–352.
17. Grieg V. *Inside Ballet Technique*. Highstown, NJ: Princeton Book; 1944: 85.
18. Anderson J. *Ballet and Modern Dance*. 2d ed. Highstown, NJ: Princeton Book; 1992: 43.
19. Hamilton WG. Physical prerequisites for ballet dancers. *J Musculoskeletal Med*. 1986; 3: 61–69.
20. Schneider HG, King AY, Bronson JL, Miller EH. Stress injuries and developmental change of lower extremities in ballet dancers. *Radiology*. 1974; 113: 627–632.
21. Anderson J. *Ballet and Modern Dance*. 2d ed. Highstown, NJ: Princeton Book; 1992: 83.
22. Teitz C, Harrington RM, Wiley H. Pressure on the foot in pointe shoes. *Foot Ankle*. 1985; 5: 216–221.
23. Tuckman HS, Werner FW, Bayley JC. Analysis of the forefoot en pointe in the ballet dancer. *Foot Ankle*. 1991; 12: 144–148.
24. Ogilvie Harris DJ, Carr MM, Fleming PJ. The foot in ballet dancers: The importance of second toe length. *Foot Ankle Int*. 1995; 16: 144–147.
25. McCurrach I. These shoes were made for dancing. *London Times, The Times Magazine*. Saturday 6 July, 2003.
26. Albers D, Hu R, McPoil T, Cornwall MC. Comparison of foot plantar pressures during walking and en pointe. *Kinesiol Med Dance*. 1992/93; 15: 25–32.
27. Laws K. *Physics and the Art of Dance. Understanding Movement*. Oxford: Oxford University Press; 2002: xi.
28. Morton DJ. *Human Locomotion and Body Form*. Baltimore, MD: Williams and Wilkins; 1952: 21.
29. Minelti AE. Three modes of terrestial locomotion in biomechanics and biology of movement. In: Nigg BM, MacIntosh R, Mester J, eds., Champaign, IL: Human Kinetics; 2000: 77.
30. Margaria R, Cavagna GA. Human locomotion in subgravity. *Aerospace Med*. 1964; 35: 1140–1146.
31. Turner RT. Physiology of a microgravity environment. *J Appl Physiol*. 2000; 89: 840–847.
32. Nicogossian AE, Huntoon CL, Pool SM. *Space Physiology and Medicine*. 2d ed. Philadelphia: Lea and Febiger; 1989: 298.
33. Wilmore JH, Costill DL. *Physiology of Sport and Exercise*. 3d ed. Champaign, IL: Human Kinetics; 2004: 343.
34. Newton's Apple. Circus High Wire www.ktca.org Production of KTCA Twin Bites Public Television and Science Teachers Association of United States. 172 4th Street East, Saint Paul, MN.
35. Blondin. In: *Encyclopaedia Brittania, Micropaedia II*. 15th ed. Chicago: Helen Hemingway, Benton; 1975: 89.
36. Petit P. *To Reach the Clouds*. London: Faber and Faber; 2002: 191.

37. Petit P. *On the High Wire*. Toronto: Random House; 1985: 14.
38. Firewalking. In: *Encyclopaedia Britannica, Micropaedia iv*, 15th ed. 152. Chicago: Helen Hemingway, Benton; 1975.
39. Burkan T. *Dying to Live*. Twain Harte, CA: Reunion; 1984: 136.
40. Wickstrom R. *Fundamental Motor Patterns*. 2d ed. Philadelphia: Lea and Febiger; 1977: 177.
41. Davids K, Lees A, Burwitz L. Understanding and measuring co-ordination and control in kicking skills in soccer. *J Sports Sci*. 2000; 18: 703–714.
42. McMurray TP. Footballer's ankle. *J Bone Joint Surg*. 1950; 32B: 68–69.
43. Asami T, Nolte V. Analysis of powerful ball kicking. In: Matsui H, Kobogeshi K, eds. *Bomechanics viii B*. Champaign, IL: Human Kinetics; 1983: 135–140.
44. Van Dijk CN, Tol JL, Verheyen CPM. A prospective study of prognostic factors concerning the outcome of arthroscopic surgery for anterior ankle impingement. *Am J Sports Med*. 1997; 24: 737–745
45. Lees A, Nolan L. The biomechanics of soccer, a review. *J Sports Sci*. 1998; 16: 211–234.
46. Maglischo EW. *Swimming Fastest*. Champaign, IL: Human Kinetics; 2003: 175.
47. *The Penny Illustrated Paper*, London. 12 October, 1861; 1,1.

7
Amputations and Prostheses

An individual's response to partial or total loss of a limb depends, to some extent, on the age when it occurs. Children adapt rapidly but most adults stoically accept the situation and make the best of it. Those who are liberated from chronic pain are only too pleased to become mobile again. As stated by a psychiatrist, James Parkes [1],

> In the early phases he feels mutilated, empty and vulnerable; as time passes he discovers how well or badly he can cope with the new world which surrounds him, and his final view of himself depends very largely upon the place which remains to him in the world and the extent to which his abilities and experience give him an expectation of satisfactory accomplishment.

Parkes compared loss of a limb to loss of a spouse. Douglas Bader, the legless fighter pilot and distinguished Royal Air Force officer, was an outstanding example for amputees as he accepted no restrictions at all in his way of living; his secret was he would not yield [2], but then he had the accident that precipitated the loss of his limbs, one below and one above the knee when he was only twenty-one-years old.

Degree of Loss: Simple to Radical

This section deals with the sequential loss of segments of the foot and ultimately the whole foot. It serves to some extent to indicate the contribution of the parts to the whole.

Amputation of the Great Toe (Hallux)

The great toe is considered essential for normal gait and it is the toe which takes the maximum pressure (see Chapter 3). Mann et al. [3] investigated the loss of the great toe in the absence of pathology in a series of ten patients who had their amputated thumbs replaced by their big toes. Measurements with a force plate revealed significant differences compared to the normal contralateral foot. In the first half of the stance phase the centre of pressure progressed from the heel to the proximal border of the region of the metatarsal heads in both feet. The initial forward movement of the centre of pressure was constant in both feet. After reaching the heads of the metatarsals there was a consistent difference between the normal and operated feet. The normal feet demonstrated a slow but continuous forward and medial progression towards the first web space. The operated foot showed a much slower forward and medial progression towards the third metatarsal head. It was clearly demonstrated that the centre of pressure moved laterally in the operated foot. There was also evidence of wear on the lateral side of the soles of their shoes and callus formation beneath the area of the second and third metatarsal heads. Nevertheless, from a functional standpoint the patients reported little or no disability from the loss of the hallux.

Amputation of All Toes

Many surgeons have considered there is no value in preserving fixed deformed and functionless toes and have advised amputation of all toes in severe cases. This procedure leaves the main weight-bearing parts of the foot intact and does not appear to have a major effect on the power of push-off and balance. The provision of shoes of normal length with a toe block compensates for the loss of the toes and allows normal walking [4]. This type of result is supported by Condie who notes [5] that the toes are the only part of the foot whose amputation does not affect the transmission of forces from midstance to toe-off. This observation is also relevant to the question of conservation of the metatarsal heads in the treatment of the grossly deformed toes, which occur in rheumatoid arthritis as excision of the metatarsal heads is common practice.

Partial Amputations of the Foot

Some classical procedures are available. Jacques Lisfranc (1790–1847) described a tarsometatarsal amputation in 1815 (and he devised long thin scalpels to divide the ligaments that join the bases of the metatarsals [6,7]. He did not describe the fracture dislocation at the tarsometatarsal junction, which is commonly attributed to him. Francois Chopart (1743–1795) is usually given credit for an amputation through the talonavicular and calcaneocuboid joints (midtarsal joint), which are covered by a long plantar flap, but he does not appear to have formally written about it. A more recent forefoot amputation is done through the cancellous bone of the bases of the metatarsal shafts. The problem with these amputations is the loss of the forefoot lever, which generates power at the ankles during push-off and this results in slower walking with increased expenditure of energy. This has been confirmed by biomechanical studies.

Mueller et al. [8] found that diabetic patients with transmetatarsal amputations suffered a 25% reduction of the power of plantarflexion. They appeared to rely on pulling the affected leg forward with their hip flexors. This functional compensation is incomplete, for the subjects also took smaller steps and walked more slowly than controls. As would be expected, the most significant deviations from normal occur during the late stance phase, when the forefoot alone would be in contact with the ground. Custom-made full-length shoes with a total contact insole, toe filler and rocker bottom sole have been shown to improve function and decrease plantar pressures.

In another study [9] after transmetatarsal amputations, it was found that only 70% of the available static range of dorsiflexion was used when walking, compared with 90% in the intact foot. It was suggested this may have been due to loss of the lever arm provided by an intact foot, and the decreased ability of the posterior calf muscles to control the forward movement of the fixed foot from midstance to toe-off.

Disarticulation at the Ankle (Syme's Amputation)

This operation was described by James Syme (1799–1870) for injuries to the foot [10]. Renowned in his day as the most eminent surgeon in the English-speaking world, during his time in the Chair of Clinical Surgery at the University of Edinburgh (1833–1869), Syme developed and perfected many new surgical procedures. All except one are now out of date. The exception is his disarticulation-amputation through the ankle joint with preservation of the heel flap to permit weight bearing. The flare of the distal tibia and fibula are removed leaving the articular surface untouched. During a period of study in Paris, Syme learnt the technique of Chopart's midtarsal amputation. He introduced the procedure in Edinburgh in 1829 and the results convinced him of its merit. The sepsis rate following Chopart's operation was low. According to Harris [11],

> This was a demonstration of the principle that in the presence of sepsis disarticulation is a much safer procedure than amputation through muscle masses and the open medullary cavities of long bones. Articular cartilage left on the end of a bone, or the subarticular cortical plate and the network of cancellous bone deep to it, serve as barriers to the spread of infection, whereas the intermuscular and fascial planes of an amputation stump provide easy pathways for invasion by micro-organisms.

Symes' favourable impression of the merit of Chopart's disarticulation led him to apply the same principle to the ankle joint. He performed his first disarticulation of the ankle joint in 1842, 13 years after his first Chopart amputation. He did not raise flaps but saved a flap from the sole of the foot by making a transverse incision and dissected the flap from the calcaneum so that the 'dense structures provided by nature for supporting the weight of the body, might still be employed for the same purpose.' Other amputations at the ankle include the Pirogoff (1854) [12] and the Boyd [13]. These operations also leave an end-bearing stump and do not require the amputee to wear an artificial limb, but shoe fitting is a major problem.

They too depend upon the integrity of the heel pad but in addition fusion of some or all of the calcaneum to the distal articular surface of the tibia. Because of difficulties with fitting, these operations are rarely done [14]. Similarly Syme's amputation is not suitable for women because of the bulk of the prosthesis, which is readily hidden beneath a trouser leg in a man.

In children with dysplasia of the fibula, Syme's amputation is a useful procedure, especially when done just before the child walks so that it knows of no other method of walking. As the whole tibia is left intact, normal growth of the bone and surrounding soft tissues occurs so that there is no need to revise the stump. Catterall [15] reported a case of a four-year-old boy who was run down by a dray in Covent Garden, London and sustained an open crush injury of his foot. He had a Syme's amputation carried out by Lister himself. Sixty-two years later he presented at King's College Hospital with dimness of vision due to a cataract. His stump had carried him without pain or hindrance protected only by a leather 'map case' type prosthesis. He had earned his living as a coal-heaver and his only regret seemed to be that his missing foot had debarred him from active service in the First World War.

Biomechanics of Midfoot and (Syme's Amputations)

Pedobarographic measurements of the vertical component of ground reaction force and the dynamic centre of pressure were recorded for five subjects with midfoot amputations (at the proximal transmetatarsal level in four and the tarsometatarsal in one) and six with Syme's disarticulations using pedobarography. Each group showed a consistent reproducible pattern of gait. The Syme's amputees walked with a standard Canadian Syme's prosthesis and SACH (solid ankle cushion heel) foot. All the midfoot amputees walked with Oxford shoes with custom-made insoles and a toe filler.

In the Syme's amputees at heel strike the ground reaction force was concentrated at the centre of the heel. The centre of pressure passed along the midline to the centre of the prosthetic forefoot where it was concentrated at push-off. In the midfoot amputees the centre of pressure started at the lateral posterior heel and proceeded distally to the bases of the metatarsals; it then shifted medially under the base of the first metatarsal where, compared with the Syme's amputees, a relatively smaller concentration of ground reaction force occurred at push-off.

These qualitative findings may explain the decreased propulsion of the midfoot amputees compared with the Syme's amputees. The shortened residual foot decreased the lever arm at push-off. Those with ankle disarticulations wearing a prosthesis with an artificial foot have a relatively normal lever arm for push-off, which accounts for a smoother, more energy-efficient gait [16], and this may explain the apparent paradoxical increased metabolic cost of walking observed in midfoot as compared to Syme's amputees.

Calcanectomy

In situations where lesions are limited to the calcaneum only, such as infection or a tumour, partial or total calcanectomy with or without disinsertion of the tendo Achillis has a place [17]. This is a rare orthopaedic procedure.

In 1931 Gaenslen [18] reported his experience of treating osteomyelitis of the calcaneum by dividing the bone in two in the sagittal plane through a midline incision across the heel pad. The resultant scars were slightly depressed but gave no trouble (cloven heel). This is an excellent approach for resection of the bone.

Total calcanectomy causes severe instability of the forefoot and the patient needs an ankle foot orthosis permanently. Stabilisation of the forefoot is possible by fusing the tibia, the navicular, and cuboid bones, after excision of the calcaneum, talus, and malleoli. The effect of the fusion is to increase the surface area for weight bearing [17].

Prosthetic Feet

Muirhead Little in the historical section of his book, *Artificial Limbs and Amputation Stumps* [19], mentions as his first example of a prosthesis, a report by Herodotus [20] of the fifth century BC in which Hezesistratus, a seer, was taken prisoner by the Spartans and condemned to death. 'He performed a deed beyond belief. For as he was confined in stocks bound with iron, he got possession of a knife . . . he cut off the broad part of the foot and escaped.' His erstwhile captors were struck with amazement at his daring when they saw half his foot lying on the ground. He fled to Tegea. Having been cured of his wounds he procured a wooden foot. Another ancient example is a bronze artificial leg from the time of the Romans, which was found in a tomb in Capua, Italy and kept in the Museum of the Royal College of Surgeons of England in London. It was thought to belong to about 300 BC as three painted vases (red figures on a black background) lay at the feet of the skeleton [21]. Unfortunately, it was destroyed during the bombing of London during the Second World War.

It is possible to cope without a prosthesis as seen in the example of Long John Silver in *Treasure Island* by Robert Louis Stevenson. 'His left leg was cut off close by the hip, and with the left shoulder he carried a crutch, which he managed with wonderful dexterity, hopping about on it like a bird' [22].The earliest known record of a crutch is a carving executed in 2830 BC [23].

One of the oldest and simplest replacements is a peg leg. These were usually wooden. It provides good comfort in the socket because it eliminates many causes of irritation of the stump. There are numerous biomechanical drawbacks. The point of support is small so that a peg leg sinks in mud or sand. The impact of heel strike cannot be cushioned adequately because of the lack of an ankle or a knee mechanism. The forward transfer of the point of support from the heel to the metatarsal heads necessary to stabilise the knee is not possible. An above-knee amputee with a peg leg has no mechanism for a knee joint. The inability to lengthen the limb during a gait cycle leads either to a characteristic circumduction of the peg or a vaulting action on the good leg [24]. Captain Ahab in the novel, *Moby Dick*, by Herman Melville had a peg leg that had been fashioned from the polished bone of a sperm whale's jaw. He steadied himself on the quarterdeck by putting his bone leg into an auger hole bored about half an inch or so into the plank (see Figure 7.1) [25].

Prostheses involving ankle and foot joints were introduced in the eighteenth century but were complex and needed frequent adjustment and repair. Synchronous movements of the prosthetic knee and ankle were introduced by

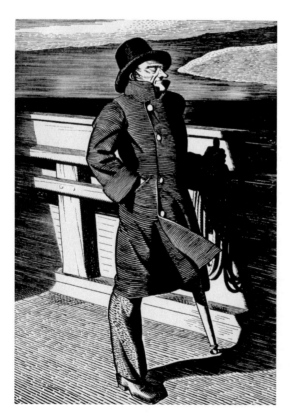

Figure 7.1. An example of a peg leg. Captain Ahab, from the novel *Moby Dick* by Herman Melville, standing on deck with his whalebone peg in a hole in the deck. (Reprinted with permission from Rockwell Kent, *Captain Ahab*, 1930, electrotype on paper, 1981, 29 ©Sterling and Francine Clark Art Institute, Williamstown, MA. Gift of J. Thomas Wilson.)

James Pott of Chelsea, London [26]. He designed a leg made of two hollow wooden cones with a steel knee joint and wooden ankle joint. Cords from the knee controlled ankle and toe movement. Because the first Marquess of Anglesey wore such a prosthesis after losing a leg at the battle of Waterloo, it became known as the Anglesey leg. With few modifications it was used by the British limb fitters until World War 1. When the knee was extended the foot was plantarflexed at the ankle by about ten degrees and when the knee was fully bent dorsiflexion of about five degrees was allowed. An Anglesey leg made of wood has the great advantage of lightness (see Figure 7.2).

The popular version of the story of the loss of the leg of the then Lord Uxbridge, Commander of the Cavalry under Wellington is that he was on horseback with the Duke of Wellington, when he was struck by grapeshot which shattered his right knee. Uxbridge exclaimed, 'By God, sir, I have lost my leg.' Wellington momentarily lowered the telescope he had been using to observe the retreating enemy and said 'By God, sir, so you have,' and resumed his survey of the victorious battlefield [27]. Lord Uxbridge was promoted to Marquess after Waterloo. A military museum at his home Plas Newydd, in Anglesey, North Wales,

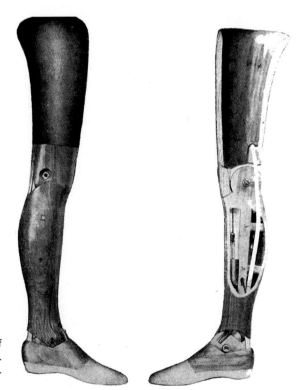

Figure 7.2. The Anglesey leg. Side view of the limb used for amputation above knee. Section showing details of construction. (Reprinted from Muirhead Little [19].)

contains a limb worn by him and a beautifully soft leather stump sock. The owner of the house where the amputation was performed, without an anaesthetic, placed Lord Uxbridge's leg in a wooden coffin and planted a weeping willow over the site where it was buried and there is still a commemorative plaque in place, which may be seen today. The Marquess of Anglesey walked daily. At the age of 67 he walked seven or eight miles and when he was 71 he danced the Polonaise at the Emperor of Russia's Winter Palace.

The modern era in the design of prosthetic feet began in 1861 when the amputee prosthetist J.E. Hanger substituted rubber bumpers for the tendon like cords that had been used as in the Anglesey limb. Over the next hundred years this and similar designs became the choice of limb fitters worldwide [28].

In the early 1950s workers at the Biomechanics Laboratory at the University of California at Berkeley developed a foot that provided a functional substitute for the single-axis foot with rubber bumpers. It is called the SACH (Solid Ankle Cushion Heel) foot. The choice of stiffness of the heel cushion, plantar flexion attitude, and alignment of the prosthesis must be carefully adjusted to suit each individual amputee. The SACH foot offers the smoothest transition from heel strike to midstance and the single-axis ankle enhances the stability of the prosthetic knee. The SACH foot is still commonly used for children's prostheses (see Figure 7.3).

An interesting variation of the SACH foot was developed by Sethi of Jaipur in India [24]. The average rural Indian does not wear shoes. He has to walk on rugged terrain, through water and mud. Urban Indian amputees do not wear shoes inside their houses, in the kitchen, and places of worship. It was decided to produce a prosthesis that did not require to be fitted with a shoe. A new design was developed. The solid wooden heel of the SACH foot was discarded. Instead two completely separate wooden blocks were used. A proximal wooden block, which approximated to the distal tibia was used for securing a carriage bolt. A distal

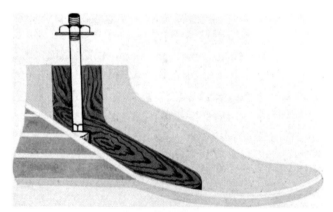

Figure 7.3. Solid ankle cushion heel (SACH foot). (Reproduced with permission from Sethi PK, Udawat MP, Kasliwal SC, et al. Vulcanized rubber foot for lower limb amputees. Prosthet Orthot Int. 1978 Dec;2(3):125–36.)

wooden block occupied the area normally represented in a foot by the distal row of tarsal bones and metatarsals. The intervening space was filled with layers of sponge rubber glued together. This could act as a universal joint with freedom of movement in all directions. Dorsi- and plantarflexion, inversion, eversion, abduction, and adduction were possible. In addition the foot as a whole could now rotate on the leg. A layer of 2 mm thick vulcanised rubber enclosed the components of the foot piece. Suitably coloured, the vulcanised rubber exterior provides a durable waterproof cover and socially acceptable cosmetic appearance.

For the sole a tougher material is used similar to that of the external facing of a motorcar tyre. Its use is restricted to the sole of the foot and can be compared to the plantar skin. The amputees feel very secure in these feet from the beginning and they require little gait training. This is thought to be a result of the large area of support.

The foot is now tailor-made in front of the user in 45 minutes. Each foot costs about 50 rupees (£0.60, Euro 0.95), whereas the below-knee prosthesis costs 150 rupees. Wearing this limb the user can work in the fields, climb trees, pull rickshaws, walk on uneven ground or even perform traditional dances (see Figures 7.4A–E). Millions of Jaipur limbs have been used in Cambodia, Vietnam, Afghanistan, and Africa [29].

A comparative study of the SACH, the Seattle foot, the first of the energy-storing feet, and Jaipur foot was carried out at The University of Liverpool in the orthopaedic department to compare their biomechanical properties using measurements of ground reaction forces. Three transtibial (below-knee) amputees participated. Each amputee was provided with an experimental limb adapted to accommodate each of three prosthetic feet. The normal foot was used as a control reference and all wore their usual limb, an Endolite patellar tendon-bearing

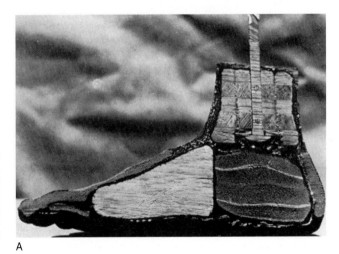

Figure 7.4. (A) Jaipur foot. Note proximal laminated wooden block. The sponge rubber universal joint consists of several layers glued together. The area corresponding to the tarsals and metatarsals is occupied by a single wooden block.

A

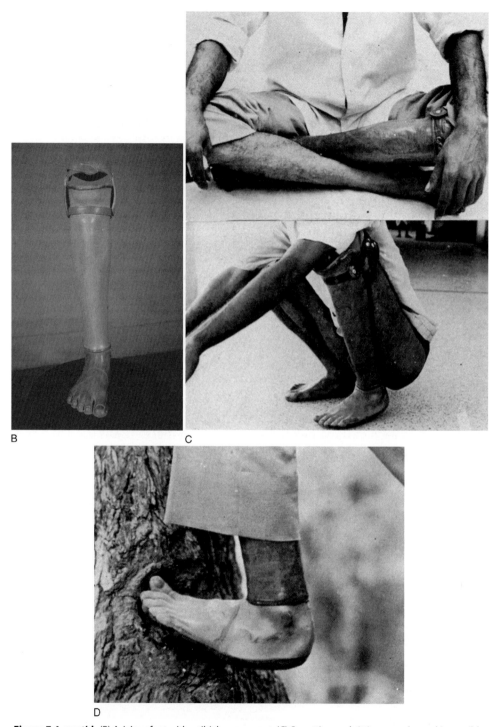

Figure 7.4. cont'd (B) A Jaipur foot with a tibial component. (C) Squatting and sitting cross-legged is possible. (D) Climbing a tree.

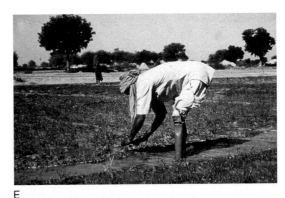

Figure 7.4. cont'd (E) Working in a rice field. (Parts A, C, D and E: Reproduced with permission from Sethi PK, Udawat MP, Kasliwal SC, et al. Vulcanized rubber foot for lower limb amputees. Prosthet Orthot Int. 1978 Dec;2(3):125–36.)

E

prosthesis with a soft prosthetic liner and Quantum foot as a terminal device during control trials. The ground reaction force was measured using a Kistler force plate. Six variables from the vertical and anteroposterior components of ground reaction forces were measured. Analysis showed that the normal foot generates significantly larger ground reaction forces than the prosthetic foot. The shock absorption capacity of the SACH foot was found to be better when compared with the other two feet, but the Jaipur foot allowed a more natural gait and was closer in performance to the normal foot [30]. Significantly less ground reaction forces are generated on the amputated side. Amputees land more softly on the prosthetic foot probably because they feel less secure than with an artificial limb as compared to a normal leg and therefore load it cautiously. The increased stresses on the normal side result in an asymmetrical gait which is consistent with previous observations that at best a normal gait in an amputee can be described as asymmetrical, having below normal acceleration and deceleration on the prosthetic side [31]. The discrepancy of weight bearing in amputees can be reduced by biofeedback training to make the best use of the body's own biological mechanisms to improve function [32].

Further detail was provided by repeating the above investigation using an EMED-SF foot pressure measurement system (see Chapter 5) [33]. It was found that the characteristics of the Seattle foot most closely resembled those of the distribution of plantar pressure in the normal foot, followed by the SACH, and then the Jaipur foot. The most important differences in plantar pressure distribution between the prosthetic feet and the normal foot were an increase in midfoot loading (140% in the Jaipur foot) and a decrease in the area of the 'toes'.

Energy Return Feet

The Seattle prosthetic foot was developed to improve the quality of life for amputees so that they could participate in sport. Until the early 1980s the feet that were fitted for amputees were only designed for walking. It was decided to design and develop an energy-storing ankle–foot unit. The first prototype foot employed a system of layered leaf spring, of a reinforced fibreglass construction, to store the energy generated during initial loading of the foot and to release this during push-off thus simulating the normal activity of the gastrocnemius and soleus muscles [34].

At about the same time an independent collaboration between a plastics engineer Dale Albildskov and a young research prosthetist, amputee Van Phillips, resulted in the creation of the Flex-Foot. This lightweight carbon fibre structure offers a radically different approach. The carbon fibre was cut into an L-shaped foot attached to a sole below and a prosthetic socket above. It simulated the spring action of the normal foot (see Chapter 3). Ultra-high-pressure, high-temperature moulding ensures the greatest strength-to-weight ratio. The chief restriction is that a minimum of five inches is required from the end of the residual limb to the floor, and seven inches or more is preferred. Unlike other prostheses the Flex-Foot uses the entire distance distal to the socket for function. Because it stores energy throughout its entire length rather than just within a four-inch keel, this results in a very resilient component. With the weight concentrated at the distal end the limb swings as if it were a sledgehammer. Even if the Flex-Foot prosthesis weighs nearly as much as a conventional limb, the patient finds it easier to use and perceives it as 'light' [35]. The mechanical concept is of a cantilevered spring, which will absorb energy during the early and midstance phases of loading and return energy in later stance phase. This pattern of foot has now been used for amputees of all levels of activity, but is most popular with amputee athletes.

In a study to determine and compare the kinematics of the sound and prosthetic limb in four of the world's best unilateral amputee sprinters, all wore patellar tendon-bearing sockets with a Flex-Foot Modular III attachment. The kinematics of the prosthetic limb were similar to those of the sound limb. All individuals achieved an 'up-on-the-toes' gait typical of sprinting in the able-bodied [36].

Since the use of the carbon fibre prosthesis 1.5 seconds has been taken off the time for 100 metres. Marion Shirley, the 100 metre champion in the Paralympics in Sydney, won in 11.09 seconds, and subsequently ran 10.97 seconds in the Utah State Summer Games, where he competed with able-bodied competition; see Figures 7.5A-C. Technological developments make it conceivable that in the future amputees may run faster than able-bodied athletes. It is interesting to note that because of the varying grades of limb now available, having run a fast 100 metres race the runner will limp off the track as the spring in the Flex-Foot is too strong for normal walking, and quickly put on a more accommodating foot for other activities.

Stiffness and hysteresis are important in the analysis of the function of artificial feet (hysteresis is the loss of energy as a part of the total energy of deformation). When dynamic response feet of varying types were tested at constant strain and

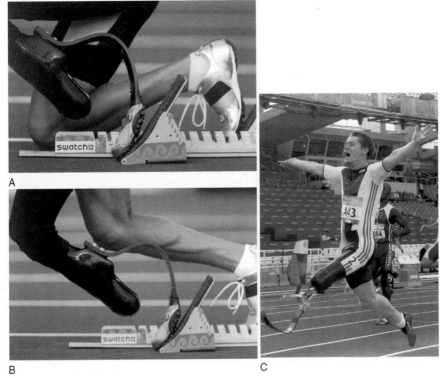

A

B   C

Figure 7.5. (A) Positioning in the starting block with a carbon fibre prosthesis. (B) Nearly ready for take off. (c) Hugo Czyz winning the 200 metres race at the Paralympics wearing a carbon fibre prosthesis. (Figures 7.5A,B reprinted with permission from Getty Images, Brian Bahr.)

in cyclical tests on an Instron Materials Testing Machine, the loss of energy varied and the least amount occurred in the Flex-Foot. Results for energy loss and hysteresis were similar [37]. A human foot is capable of strong strain energy and it returns that energy in the form of an elastic recoil. Alexander et al. [38] suggest the latter is in the range of 22 ± 1%. In contrast the Flex-Foot when tested as above showed only a 10% loss of energy because it is more elastic than the viscoelastic ligamentous tissues of the normal foot. In all biological materials the viscous element causes the stress developed to be partly dependent on the rate of strain and the strain itself to change with time [39].

With the excellent prostheses now available for below-knee amputees the place of partial foot and even Syme's amputations need to be carefully considered when faced with cases of trauma in young active subjects. Although it is natural for a surgeon to want to preserve as much of a foot as possible, the functional outcome of partial foot amputations is far less useful than can be provided by a successful below-knee operation fitted with a modern prosthesis.

Phantom Limb

This troublesome feature was known to Ambrose Paré (1510–1590), the famous French surgeon who introduced the ligature to amputation surgery and abandoned the red-hot cautery for control of haemorrhage. He wrote, 'Patients imagine that they have their members yet entire, and yet doe complain thereof (which I imagine to come to passé, for that the cut nerves retire themselves towards their originall and thereby cause a paine like to convulsions)' [40]. He recommends an ointment to be applied on 'the spine of the back and all the affected part for relief of pain.'

Rene Descartes (1569–1605), the French philosopher, mathematician, and scientist, who conceived of the pain system as a straight channel from the skin to the brain, according to Walther Riese, referred in his writing to the various pains of which a girl complained whose arm had been amputated from the elbow. The pains were felt sometimes in one finger of the hand that had been amputated and sometimes in another, just as in a phantom limb. He offered the explanantion that

The nerves which before stretched downwards from the brain to the hand and then terminated in the arm close to the elbow, were there moved in the same way as they required to be moved before in the hand for the purpose of impressing on the mind residing in the brain the sensation of pain in this or that finger.

He concluded that the pain of the hand was in fact felt in the brain [41].

In *Moby Dick* by Herman Melville published in 1851 [25], Captain Ahab in a conversation with the carpenter who is making him a new peg leg (see Figure 7.1) says 'when I come to mount this leg thou makest, I shall nevertheless feel another leg in the same identical place with it; that is, carpenter, my old lost leg; the flesh and blood one I mean. . . . I still feel the smart of my crushed leg, though it be now so long dissolved.' It is clear that the phenomenon of phantom limb was recognised long before the term was introduced by Silas Weir Mitchell (1829–1914), the leading American neurologist of his time. With George Read Morehouse and William W Kean, he studied gunshot and other injuries of the peripheral nerves sustained during the Civil War.

Nearly every man who loses a limb carries about with him a constant or inconstant phantom of the missing member, a sensory ghost of that much of himself, and sometimes a most inconvenient presence, faintly felt at times but ready to be called up to his perception by a blow, a touch or a change of wind. . . .

Very many have a constant sense of the existence of the limb, a consciousness even more than exists for the remaining member. 'If' says one 'I should say I am more sure of the leg which aint than the one which are, I guess I should be about correct. . . .

Silas Weir Mitchell [42]

It is likely that central representation of the limb survives after amputation and is responsible for the illusion. Patients frequently complain that the phantom is painful and as many as 70% of phantoms remain painful 25 years after loss of the limb. The origin of phantom pain is no less mysterious than the origin of phantoms themselves [43].

Phantoms are seen far less often in early childhood. Perhaps in young children there has not been enough time for the body image to consolidate [44]. Stump pathology (e.g., scarring and neuromas) influence both the vividness and duration of the phantom. Silas Weir Mitchell too noted that a phantom fades more rapidly if the stump heals quickly and well [45].

A variety of methods has been tried to relieve phantom pain which range from analgesic drugs to transcutaneous nerve stimulators and neurosurgical procedures. A promising new technique using a 'virtual reality box' has been introduced by Ramachandran [46]. This is made by placing a vertical mirror inside a cardboard box with the roof of the box removed. The front of the box has two holes through which the patient inserts his good and his phantom limb. The patient when looking at the reflection of his normal limb has an illusion he has two limbs and he is seeing his phantom. If he sends motor commands to both limbs he will think his phantom limb has been resurrected and is obeying his commands. Involuntary painful spasms in the phantom limb have been relieved using this technique. Studies using PET (positron emission tomography) and magnetic resonance imaging suggested there is a considerable amount of latent plasticity even in the adult human brain. For example, precisely organised new pathways, bridging the two cerebral hemispheres can emerge in less than three weeks [46].

Work on phantom limbs and their neural basis has progressed at a rapid pace recently. It is now clear that this phenomenon provides a valuable experimental opportunity to investigate how new connections emerge in the adult human brain; how information from different sensory modalities (e.g., touch, proprioception, and vision) interact and how the brain continuously updates its model of reality in response to novel sensory impulses [43].

References

1. Parkes CN. Psycho-social transitions: Comparison between reactions to loss of a limb and loss of a spouse. *Brit J Psychiatry.* 1975; 127: 204–210.
2. Brickhill P. *Reach for the Sky. The Story of Douglas Bader – Hero of the Battle of Britain.* London: Cassell; 1954.
3. Mann RA, Poppen NK, O'Konski M. Amputation of the great toe. *Clin Orthopaed Related Res.* 1988; 226: 192–205.
4. Flint M, Sweetnam R. Amputation of all toes. *J Bone Joint Surg.* 1960; 42B: 90–94.
5. Condie DW. Biomechanical and prosthetic considerations. In: Murdoch G, Bennett Wilson, A, eds. *Amputation Surgical Practice and Patient Management.* Oxford: Butterworth. Heinemann; 1996: 13.
6. Lisfranc J. Nouvelle methode operatour pour l'amputation partiella du pied dans son articulation tarso-metatarsienne; methode precedes les nombreuses modifications qu'a subies celle de Chopart. Paris: Gabon; 1815.

7. Kirkup J. Personal communication about Lisfranc's knives.

8. Mueller MJ, Salsich GB, Bastian AJ. Differences in the gait characteristics of people with diabetes and tarsometatarsal amputation compared with age matched controls. *Gait Posture*. 1998; 7: 200–206.

9. Garbalosa JC, Cavanagh PR, Wu G, Ulbrecht, JS, Becker MB, Alexander JF, Campbell JH. Foot function in diabetic patients after partial amputation. *Foot Ankle Int*. 1996; 17: 43–48.

10. Syme J. Amputation at the ankle joint. *London Edinburgh Monthly J*. 1843; XXXVI: 93–96.

11. Harris RI. History and development of Syme's amputation. *Artif Limbs*. 1961; 6: 4–43.

12. Pirogoff NI. *Voyenno Med J St.Petersburg lxiii, 2 sect.*, 1854; 83–100

13. Boyd HB. Amputation of the foot with calcaneo-tibia arthrodesis. *J Bone Joint Surg*. 1939; 21: 997–1000.

14. English E. Syme's amputation. In: Kostuik JP, Gillespie R, eds. *Amputation Surgery and Rehabilitation*. New York: Churchill Livington; 1981: 81.

15. Catterall RCF. Syme's amputation by Joseph Lister after sixty six years. *J Bone Joint* Surgery. 1967; 49: 144–145.

16. Pinzur MS, Wolf B, Harvey RM. Walking pattern of midfoot and ankle disarticulation amputees. *Foot Ankle Int*. 1997; 18: 635–638.

17. Baumgartner R. Partial foot amputations. In: Murdoch G, Bennett Wilson A, eds. *Amputation Surgical Practice and Patient Management*. Oxford: Butterworth Heinemann; 1996:101.

18. Gaenslen FJ. Split heel approach in osteomyelitis of os calcis. *J Bone Joint Surg*. 1931; 13: 759–792.

19. Muirhead Little E. *Artificial Limbs and Amputation Stumps*. London: HK Lewis; 1922: 1.

20. Herodotus. Translated by Cary HF. London: George Bell and Sons; 1908: 559.

21. MacDonald J. The history of artificial limbs. *Am J Surg*. 1905; 19: 76–82.

22. Stevenson RL. *Treasure Island*. New York: Charles Scribner's Sons; 1901: 55.

23. Epstein S. Art history and the crutch. *Ann Med* Hist. 1937; 9: 304–313.

24. Sethi PK, Udawot MP, Kasliwal SC, Chandra R. Vulcanised rubber foot for lower limb amputees. *Prosthet Orthot Int*. 1978; 2: 125–136.

25. Melville H. *Moby Dick*. New York: Modern Library; 2000; pegleg: 230, phantom limb: 677.

26. Rang M, Thompson, GH. History of amputations and prostheses. In: Kostuick JP, Gillespie R, eds. *Amputation Surgery and Rehabilitation*. New York: Churchill Livingston; 1981:11.

27. The Marquess of Anglesey. *One-leg. The Life and Letters of Henry William Paget, First Marquess of Anglesey, by the present Marquess of Anglesey*, London: Leo Cooper; 1996: 149.

28. Radcliffe CW. Prosthetics. In: *Human Walking*. Rose J, Gamble JG, eds. Baltimore, MD: Williams and Wilkins; 1994: 165–200.

29. South Asian theme issue, No mean feet. Interview with Singhal, D, Nudny, S. *Brit Med J*. 2004; 328: 789.

30. Arya AP, Lees A, Nirula HC, Klenerman L. A biomechanical comparison of the SACH, Seattle and Jaipur feet using ground reaction forces. *Prosthet Orthot Int*. 1995; 19: 37–45.

31. Van Leeuwen JL, Speth LA, Deanen HA. Shock absorption of below knee prostheses; A comparison between the SACH and multiflex foot. *J Bomech*. 1990; 23: 441–446.

32. Quinlivin DH. Weight distribution in below-knee amputees. In: *Proceedings of the annual scientific meeting of International Society of Prosthetics and Orthotics*, Blackpool, United Kingdom, 9–11 February 1994; 31.

33. Nyska M, Shabat S, Arys A, McCabe C, Linze K, Klenerman L. A comparative study of different below-knee prostheses by dynamic foot pressure analysis. *Int J Rehab Res*. 2002; 25: 341–344.

34. Burgess EM, Hittenberger DA, Forsgren SM, Lindh DV. The Seattle prosthetic foot – A design for active sports: Preliminary studies. *Orthot Prosthet*. 1983; 37: 25–31.

35. Michael J. Energy storing feet: A clinical comparison. *Clin Prosthet Orthot*. (1987). 11: 154–168.

36. Buckley JG. Sprint kinematics of athletes with lower-limb amputations. *Arch Phys Med Rehab.* 1999; 80: 501–508.
37. Geil MD. Energy loss of stiffness properties of dynamic elastic response feet. *J Prosthet Orthot.* 2001; 13: 70–73.
38. Ker RF, Bennett MB, Bilby SR, Kester RC, Alexander McNeill R.. The spring in the arch of the human foot. *Nature.* 1987; 325: 147–149.
39. Cochran GVB. A primer of orthopaedic biomechanics. New York: Churchill Livingston; 1982: 91.
40. The Apologie and Treatise of Ambroise Paré. Keynes G, Ed. London: Falcon Educational; 1951: 154.
41. Riese W. Descartes' ideas of brain function. In: Poynter FNL, ed. *The Brain and Its Functions.* Oxford: Blackwell Scientific; 1958:115–134.
42. Mitchell SW. *Injuries of Nerves and Their Consequences.* Philadelphia J. B. Lippincott; 1872: 348.
43. Ramachandran VS, Hirstein W. The perception of phantom limbs. The D. O. Hebb lecture. *Brain.* 1998; 121: 1603–1630.
44. Simmel M. The reality of phantom sensations. *Social Res.* 1962; 29: 337–356.
45. Sutherland S. Nerves and nerve injuries. London: E. and S. Livingstone; 1968: 456.
46. Ramachandran VS, Rogers-Ramachandran D, Synaesthesia in phantom limbs induced with mirrors. *Proc Roy Soc London.* 1996; 264: 437–444.

Index